**An Inspiring Story of a Husband & Wife
Winning the Battle Against Cancer Together**

Stronger
with
Two

BARI ROBERTS ROSS

Stronger with Two

The Inspiring True Story of a Husband & Wife Winning the Battle Against Cancer Together

© 2020 Bari Roberts Ross

ISSN: 978-1-950681-10-5

Cover and Interior Design by AugustPride, LLC
Back Cover Photo: Jack Kearse, Emory University

ILLUMINATION Press
1100Peachtree Street
Suite 250
Atlanta, Georgia 30309
United States

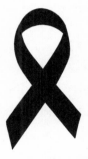

ACKNOWLEDGEMENTS

I wake up every day with an "attitude of gratitude." Before my feet touch the floor, I thank God for my journey and for opportunities to serve. I am also thankful for the many angels he has placed on my path. I am most grateful for the two angels he allowed me to birth, my daughters Brooke Richards and Staci Fowler. They married two angels that I call my sons, Stephen and Christian. I am forever blessed to have David, Bria and Skyelar as my grandchildren who uplift me with the sound of their voices calling me "Mema." To my "Grand-dog Kingston" thank you for your protection and loyalty.

One thing I know for sure, "family is everything." Thank you to my mother, father and stepmother who gave me the best of what they had. To my sister Traci and my brother Tim what a privilege to have shared our parents with you. To my "sister-friend" Deborah Mooreman-Williams you are a special angel that has been with me since middle school.

To Regenia and Jerone Vessels you became my angels the day Charles and I got married and have steadfastly flown by our side. To my sisters-in-laws Polly Morgan, Shirley Chambliss, Odell Jones, Ella

Mae Cook and Arlene Roberts thank you for your love and caregiving in our darkest days.

Reverend Robert and First Lady Odessa Perry and my Union Baptist Church family, Pastor Gregory and First Lady Libby Pollard and the Enon Baptist Church family and Bishop Todd and Pastor Linda Emerson and the House of Joy. I am forever grateful for your prayers, support and tender mercies to us.

To my Atlanta Sisterhood -Tauheedah Amon-Ra, Maria Ayree, Desiree Sanchez, Hasina Grimball, Roberta Davy, Earline Gibbs, Thebither Michels, Joanne Kenner, Marcia Carpenter, Jennifer Reid, Sharon Jones, Britta Tabor, Thelema Martin, Bettie Jones, June Anderson, Dr. Millicent Henry, Lois Ford, Monica Davis:

My Phoenix Sisterhood-Beverly Brooks Carroll, Fatimah Halim, Diana Gregory, Miasia Pasha, Yvette Craddock, Cheryl Lynne Jones, Tonya Allen, Veronica Clark, Nazalah Hassan, Maudelle Terry, Marion Johnston, Lebertha Umbreit, Dawn Agent and Kenyatta Turner. Thank you for your enduring friendship.

Special thanks to Laverne Jones for all you have quietly guided me through in our many years of friendship and to Michelle Graves for you wonderful She'ology Organic products that not only helped heal my radiation burns but also touched my heart. Wanda Wright, Lasana Hotep, Rashaunda and Melvin Lugrand you are very special to my heart and are my "bonus children" because you choose to call me "Momma".

Much love and honor to three women who I call Mother and who love me like a daughter, Yvonne Peek, Blanche Sumpter and Mary Stanley.

Thank you Lawanda Long and Michael Anderson for praying with me as I started my journey on this book. Dorothy Randall Gray thank you for introducing me to my writing Muse many years ago. Much Gratitude to Benecia Ponder and Illumination Press for helping me bring my dream for this book into reality.

To my mentor who fought cancer twice and is now at rest, I was blessed that you inspired me to move forward no matter how challenging the battle, thank you forever Julie Whitehead.

To the amazing doctors, nurses and staff at Emory Healthcare-Winship Cancer Institute words cannot express Charles and my gratitude for your compassion and dedication to our not just surviving but thriving after cancer.

To my phenomenal husband I am comforted daily by your strength, courage and love.

TABLE OF CONTENTS

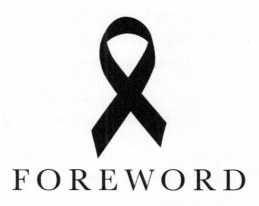

FOREWORD

I never thought that my role as a caregiver would happen the way it did. I was living, working in New York. My mother was enjoying her retirement in Alabama. Suddenly, everything changed. My mother was scheduled to have a tumor removed and after what seemed like a successful surgery, my mother was told that she had Stage 4 Large T-Cell Lymphoma.

I felt guilty that I was unable to be by my mother's side, especially as she grappled with this new reality. Family, friends, and people in our communities rallied around us, encouraging us to stay strong and to pray.

It was painfully obvious that my mother, who could barely walk, would need around the clock care. The question was—who would help my mother recover? Until this question was answered, my mother's cousin and her partner swooped in, transferring her to Emory Hospital in Atlanta, Georgia. My brother, prepping for a move out of the country, rushed to be by my mother's side.

These were not long-term commitments. I knew a hard decision

1

needed to be made. With my husband's blessing, we decided that it would be best for me to help. I packed one suitcase and temporarily relocated to Georgia to become my mother's caregiver.

Life as a caregiver was entering uncharted territory. I didn't understand the magnitude of what I was undertaking.

From uprooting my mother, to pushing her wheelchair, to getting her dressed, preparing her meals, paying her bills, attending doctor's appointments and week-long chemotherapy sessions, caregiving kept me on my toes. The hardest part was reading the paperwork and trying to understand what the doctors were saying.

The moment I was introduced to Bari and, her husband Charles, I knew it had to be divine intervention. Bari and Charles became a signal of hope and perseverance. Bari eased my fears, explaining medical terminology in a way that kept me from feeling overwhelmed. Bari's genuine spirt offered reassurance that things would be okay—I would have to believe this with every bone in my body. And I did.

My mom survived. I think every caregiver needs support from family, friends, their community or, in my case, a knowledgeable advocate like Bari because the act of caregiving cannot be something you do alone.

- Kadiyah Lodge -

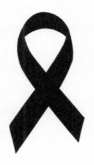

PROLOGUE

On October 26, 2008, Charles and I were looking forward to celebrating our sixth anniversary. Until a few months prior, we were still behaving like young newlyweds, though we were certainly firmly planted in middle-age. It was both of our second marriages after many years of being single. We had changed our lives to start anew. A new city, Phoenix, Arizona, a new house, a new small restaurant and what was beginning to look like a new health challenge.

We spent months planning a cruise to the Western Caribbean for our anniversary, but Charles was in bed resting, suffering from exhaustion. He refused to go to the doctor.

"Honey, I'm just tired. My energy is low, and I feel like I have the flu. I just had my annual physical two months ago and everything looked good. I don't need to go to the doctor for this. I just want to rest."

"Charles, what about that bruise on your leg? You hit it against a counter three weeks ago and it doesn't seem to be healing. I think it needs to be looked at by your doctor."

"I want to give it a little more time to heal itself. It doesn't hurt. Right now, I just want to sleep and when I get up maybe we can to Popo's for a good Mexican dinner and you can have your favorite mango margarita."

We didn't go to dinner. His malaise worsened over the next few days. I called his doctor to make an appointment for the earliest availability which was two weeks later. During that two weeks, Charles was barely able to drag himself out of bed for more than four hours a day. He was losing weight and struggled to stand in the shower. The doctor diagnosed him with strep throat and gave him a ten-day supply of antibiotics. He scheduled another appointment for two weeks later. We were relieved that it was something as common as strep.

Ten days later, Charles was not feeling any better; he now had swellings under his arms and in his groin. When he saw the doctor, the diagnosis changed from strep to a lymph node infection. The doctor asked him if we had been out of the country or if I had any symptoms. Charles said no. So, the doctor prescribed a stronger antibiotic for five more days.

Things did not improve—not only were there swellings, but they started to hurt. Charles went back to the doctor for blood tests. A few days later, his doctor said that his white blood cells were elevated and that he was referring him to an Ear, Nose and Throat doctor. He couldn't schedule an appointment for almost three weeks.

In early February, Charles' sister, Katie, lost her battle with colorectal cancer. Charles announced, "I am going to Virginia for a week to attend her memorial service and spend time with my family."

I believed that was a good sign that he was going to travel. I also thought he would share with his family that we were struggling and give them some idea of his illness. He did neither. He mentioned to them he had a recurring infection and led them to believe everything in Phoenix was the same as when they had visited a year prior.

When Charles returned from Virginia the following Sunday, I met him at the airport, and he looked haggard and tired. He was bent over at the waist and could barely hold his carry-on.

Since our restaurant was closed every Monday, I was able to stay home and take care of him. The next day, Charles said he felt strong enough to go to the doctor by himself. I went to the restaurant. After closing, I rushed home to hear what the doctor said. Charles was sitting on the side of the bed. It was apparent he hadn't received good news.

"The doctor dropped a scope down my throat and said, 'this doesn't look good, Mr. Ross.' Honey, I fainted. He wants to see us in his office on Thursday afternoon."

I ran to the computer and looked up what kind of scope a doctor could use to determine something "didn't look good" and to understand what that "something" could be. Based on his other symptoms and his age, the choices were myriad. We had to wait another forty-eight hours to get an answer.

We arrived at the appointment early. As I looked around the office, I found comfort that none of the waiting patients seemed visibly sick. When they called us to the examination room, Charles was unsteady on his feet, I held his arm and led him down the hall.

"Mr. Ross, your blood tests are very concerning, along with your swollen lymph nodes. I've scheduled you for a biopsy of the lymph node under your chin next Friday morning. The blood tests rule out an infection, but I don't have a diagnosis. I'm certain the biopsy will give a clearer picture."

"Ok doctor, but what about my wife? She has swelling behind her right ear."

My brain was processing what the doctor said. "Honey, what are you talking about? I don't have any swelling. I'm fine."

"I saw it last night when you were sleep, and I thought maybe I gave you my infection. But since the doctor said it's not an infection, I want him to look at you."

I ran my hand over the area behind my ear and felt a slight swelling about the size of a grape. The doctor came over and looked at my neck and said, "Mrs. Ross, ask my receptionist to make an appointment for you tomorrow."

I was confident that we had something contagious and that perhaps once I was tested, Charles wouldn't need a biopsy.

On the drive home, I wanted to ask Charles why he waited to tell me about my neck at the doctor's office, but he was asleep. Once we were home, neither of us could eat. Charles went to bed, and I went to WebMD. I didn't know what to look for, so I soon gave up and watched television until I fell asleep.

* * *

I arrived at my appointment with no worries. After checking me in, the nurse performed the perfunctory weight, temperature, and blood pressure measurements. When she finished, the doctor was right behind her. He looked at my medical history and examined my neck.

"Mrs. Ross, I want to do what is called a fine needle biopsy on that swelling behind your ear. I will numb the area, take a piece and send it to the lab."

"I don't recall Charles telling me that you did this to him."

"I didn't do this to him. I did different tests on him. I don't think you two have the same thing," he spoke softly as he prepared his instruments.

"I also made an appointment for you to have a Cat Scan."

I didn't flinch as he stuck me with the first needle to numb the area. My mind was racing in different directions with the words, "not the same thing."

I never felt the second needle, and within minutes it was over. He told me to expect a call from his office in a couple of days.

I stopped at the store and grabbed the ice cream. Charles was sleep and didn't move when I came in. I turned on the computer and when the search bar appeared, I typed, "fine needle biopsy." I read the results:

"A needle biopsy may reveal whether a mass or lump is a cyst, an infection, a benign tumor or cancer.

Analysis from a needle biopsy can help doctors determine what germs are causing an infection so that the most effective medications can be prescribed."

My eyes went directly to the second definition of how it was useful in diagnosing an infection. I relaxed and prepared a light dinner. When Charles woke, I told him about the appointment, "That's good, I hope that he can get to the bottom of this because I am feeling weaker every day."

"I think we're getting close to a diagnosis. I trust this doctor. I'm going to give you your ice cream before dinner. How does that sound?"

"You know how to make me feel good. Two scoops and a kiss, then I'll feel even better."

Two days later, I got a call from the doctor's office for an appointment the following day. I was impressed with the turn-around time.

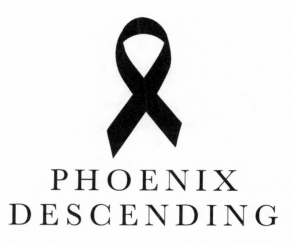

PHOENIX DESCENDING

April 2009. The 104-degree oven-like heat rose from the ground, baking everything in its path.

I stepped out of my car and headed to the doctor's office for the third time in a week. I was hoping for a mist system around the entrance to give me a few seconds of relief before entering the building. There was no mist, but as the door opened, a burst of cold air greeted me, enough to give me a chance to catch a refreshing breath.

As I waited for the elevator, my exterior was calm, but my mind was racing. When I was in high school, one of my teachers would start every class, "Define the problem, solve the problem." She taught us to gather all the facts, not to jump to any conclusions, and then work it through to the solution.

I was holding on to that wisdom.

When I arrived in the office, only one person was sitting in the waiting area. It wasn't long before the nurse was leading me down the dimly lit hall to the last room.

"Have a seat on the couch, and the doctor will be with you momentarily," she said, placing a box of Kleenex next to me.

I had a bottle of water in my purse. It was warm, but my throat was parched. I took a few sips and exhaled a sigh.

I heard the doctor chatting and laughing with someone down the hall, but as he stood outside of the door rustling the papers in my file, his laughter stopped.

"Good afternoon, Mrs. Ross."

I smiled weakly and nodded. My mouth was so dry that I couldn't speak.

"I have some bad news for you. The pathology report and the Cat Scan show that you have Squamous Cell Cancer in your right tonsil, and it has metastasized to your lymph nodes. This is a very aggressive cancer, and you need treatment as soon as possible," the doctor explained as he moved the box of Kleenex closer to me.

I pushed it back.

Now was not the time for me to cry. I was using everything in me to understand his definition of the problem. I was confused because other than a small swelling below my right earlobe, I had no other symptoms to indicate that there was anything wrong with my health.

"So, what are we going to do about it?" I asked to gather as much information as possible.

He pulled papers out of the file.

"I looked up a few things before you arrived. The first person I would highly recommend for your type of advanced cancer is a world renown doctor at the Mayo Clinic; however, he doesn't take your insurance. The second person is a good friend of mine and has experience with what you have, but he doesn't take your insurance either."

I was getting annoyed. I sat still and let him continue.

"I found someone in the Physician's Directory who takes your insurance. I don't know much about him. My secretary called his office, and he can see you in six weeks."

I slowly repeated his words, "This first and best doctor who would give me a good chance of beating this doesn't take my insurance, neither does the second best in the Phoenix area. You don't know anything about the last one, except that he takes my insurance and he can't see me for six weeks, while I have rapidly growing metastatic cancer."

He pushed the Kleenex box towards me again and said: "Yes, that is correct."

I pushed the Kleenex box to the side realizing that he had defined the problem but had no credible solution.

I took a deep breath and blew out my frustration.

"You are having an insurance conversation. I need a 'save Bari's life' conversation. Right now, it seems our conversations are running parallel and they aren't meeting at any point."

He looked out the window towards the shimmering White Tank Mountains.

"So, what do you want to do?" he asked me.

Apparently, this doctor didn't have the solutions I needed.

"Thank you for your time and the diagnosis, but I don't see a way forward here. Please give me my pathology report and CT Scan. I will sign any papers to release you from any further action on my behalf. Continue to work with my husband. I will see you at his appointment on Friday."

He shook my hand, wished me luck, and left the room. I looked out the window at the mountains. It was midday, and the sun was at an angle that made them seem snowcapped, despite the one hundred plus temperature.

I put the box of Kleenex in the cabinet, stopped by the front desk, took my medical reports, and walked out the door toward the mountain.

I opened the car door. The heat jumped out and wrapped itself around me like a straitjacket. I couldn't breathe and realized that I was having a panic attack. I refused to surrender to the fear. I needed a clear, logical mind to solve the problem.

I turned the air condition to its highest level. I opened the envelope and read the pathology report for myself. The language was foreign, but there were three key words that I understood: Cancer, Metastatic, Advanced Stage.

"I need a second opinion. This may be a big mistake," I thought.

"But if it isn't, what am I going to do?"

I took out the CT scan and it looked like an x-ray broken into hundreds of puzzle pieces. I held it up to the light but I couldn't make any sense of it. I certainly couldn't see cancer. I couldn't even make out a neck, a tongue, or any distinct body part. I sat there for a while and let the cold air wash over me. I couldn't go home and tell Charles this news when I didn't have a plan.

I grabbed my cellphone and pushed the first number on speed dial. My daughter, Brooke, answered the phone cheerily.

"Hi Mommy, how are you? I hope you didn't call to rub in how wonderful the weather is in Phoenix. It's been raining here in Atlanta for the last week."

"Brooke are you at work?" I whispered.

"Yes... Why? What's wrong? Did they find out what's going on with Papa Charles?"

"No, they still don't know what is wrong with Charles, but I have some bad news... concerning me."

I heard her breath escape her body, but before she could say anything I blurted out, "I am sitting outside of the doctor's office with a pathology report and a CT Scan that says I have cancer coming out of my right tonsil, and it has spread to my lymph nodes."

I repeated to her what the doctor said about the best doctors not taking my insurance, and that the third doctor couldn't see me for six weeks. Brooke was at work at the premier hospital in Atlanta.

"Mommy, go to the nearest Staples and fax me your pathology report, then go to FedEx and overnight me the CT Scan. Don't worry, I'll get you answers once I get the information."

I drove out of the parking lot and took one more look at the now shadowy mountain in the rearview mirror. Within minutes I arrived at Staples and paced in line waiting for the fax machine. When it was available, I tried to take the pathology report out of the envelope, but my hands were shaking. It felt like an enormous task. I stepped back and let the next person in line use the machine. I went to the ladies' room and splashed cold water on my face and willed myself not to fall apart.

I walked straight to the machine, inserted the dollar, and entered the phone number. I heard the familiar gurgling sound and high beep that a fax machine makes as it connects.

When the fax submission was complete, I felt a sense of relief. I could envision Brooke standing at the other end, grabbing and reading each sheet as it came through.

Brooke called. She still sounded professional but somber. We knew that a time to cry was coming but now was not the moment.

"Mommy, this is very serious. I took your report to the doctor that I work for, and he said 'get your mother on a plane tonight and get her here tomorrow.' I have made a reservation for you on the red-eye to leave Phoenix at 10:30 tonight and arrive in Atlanta at 5:55 in the morning."

I was in a state of dread because of what her doctor said and a state of relief that my daughter took control of the situation. I was in turmoil because I hadn't spoken to Charles. Given his uncertain health, I couldn't fly off in eight hours and leave him alone.

"Brooke, I haven't told Papa Charles anything, and I need some time to shore things up here. He is scheduled to see the Doctor on Friday for a biopsy. I'll call you back."

"Mommy, you don't have a minute to spare; you have got to get here as soon as possible!"

Brooke's voice was losing its professional tone and had the beginnings of a tremble.

I said gently, "I'll call you back soon. I promise."

I hung up so that we could maintain what was left of our composure.

I realized that I had not eaten, and the car was almost out of gas. I didn't know where I was, and panic was engulfing me like a giant wave swallows a surfer. I wanted to surrender and let the tide carry me out to sea, but I felt close enough to paddle to the shore.

I looked through my phone contacts and found Charles' sister Regenia's number. It went to voice mail. I remembered the three-hour time difference and realized she was at work.

The gas light was blinking. The last thing I needed was to get stuck by the side of the road in 110-degree temperature. I didn't have enough money to fill the tank, so I put in enough to make it home.

I looked at my phone, waiting for Regenia's name to pop up on the screen. It had only been twenty minutes, but in that time, I came up with a plan that required her help.

15

I dialed her home number and her husband, Jerry, jovially answered the phone,

"Hi, Bari. How are you and Charlie doing? I know the weather out there is dry and sunny, we are having a wet spring in Virginia."

"Jerry, I called Regenia, and I need to talk to her as soon as possible."

Those were the last coherent words I spoke. I broke down in blubbering tears as I tried to explain to him what happened in the last three hours.

When I caught my breath, he said, "She's at school but stand by. I will call her, and she will call you back in a few minutes."

When I saw her name on the screen, I breathed. I told her my diagnosis and the plans that Brooke had for me to come to Atlanta. I told her about Charles' situation and the upcoming biopsy on Friday.

"Can you come and be with Charles? I must leave for Atlanta. I feel like I am running for my life."

"I will talk to Jerry. I feel certain I'll be able to come. Hang in there."

I felt that I at least had the first steps of a plan to give us a small bit of comfort to get us through what was going to be a long, emotional night.

When I got home, Charles was asleep and didn't move when I came into the room. I went into the kitchen and poured a generous glass of cold water.

Instead of gulping the water, I sipped it and let it drizzle down my throat.

16

My throat that now had cancer.

I touched my throat; the throat that swallowed every morsel of food I have ever eaten. The throat that gave sound to every hearty laugh and every sad cry I have heaved. My throat that sung happy songs and the blues.

My throat that yelled at my daughters and spoke words of love to them. My throat that spoke in angry tones and words of kindness and encouragement to people. My throat that said its last goodbye to my mother on her deathbed. My throat that spoke proudly and, at times, swallowed my pride.

My phone rang. I grabbed it, hoping that Charles didn't hear it.

It was Regenia.

"I will be flying into Phoenix on Saturday at 11:00 am. I can stay a week. Do you guys need anything else?"

"Thank you, Regenia, I will make a reservation to leave shortly after you arrive. I will bring Charles to the airport. We will meet you in the atrium."

I called Brooke to tell her she could make flight arrangements for me after 12:30 p.m. on Saturday. I didn't want to talk long. I knew I would break down.

I had to pack. My photos were the highest priority. Everything else was replaceable; but the precious images of family members, my children, and grandchildren, of celebrations and travel were priceless. I knew instinctively my time of living in Phoenix was ending and that my work now was to ensure that my life wasn't ending, but if it was, my daughters would have the pictures.

I put a pair of sneakers, a pair of slacks, a blouse, one lightweight jacket and my favorite pair of earrings into the suitcase. I didn't want to be loaded down with "stuff." I was already carrying the burden of having cancer, and I had no idea how much heavier it would become.

I heard Charles stirring a bit in the bedroom. I waited a few minutes to gather myself. He patted the bed and asked me to sit by him. I saw how much weight he lost and how drawn his face was. His skin looked dull, and his eyes looked hollow. My heart was breaking at the thought of telling him that as healthy as I looked, there was cancer metastasizing in me. My perceived good health was a sham.

"My lovely wife, how did your visit with the doctor go?"

I reached out for his hand and held it tightly.

"It didn't go so well, Honey. The doctor said all the tests indicate that I have cancer, and that it has spread."

"Oh, my Lord!" he cried "Why? Not my wife, no, no!"

Tears streamed from my eyes as I watched him wrestle with my news, his illness, and his whys to God. I waited for him to calm down before speaking. I knew that what I was going to say next would hit him like a roundhouse punch.

"The best doctors out here don't take our insurance. I called Brooke, and she said the hospital she works at is willing to take me as a patient. I need to get there as soon as possible."

18

"You need to go to Atlanta for treatment?"

"Yes, and I'm leaving Saturday afternoon. I will be here with you Friday when you have your biopsy. Regenia will be here Saturday and she will stay with you for a week."

I looked away because the pain in his face was unbearable.

He was weeping. I saw he needed to do it privately as he sorted through the tsunami of events that was released. I stepped out of the bedroom and went to the porch and breathed in the hot air. I listened to him as he wailed and then as he softly snored before falling into sleep.

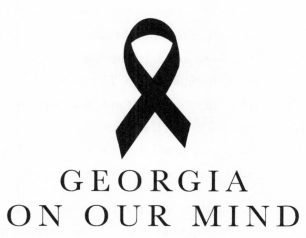

GEORGIA
ON OUR MIND

When I entered the kitchen the next morning, Charles was sitting at the table. His head was hung low, and silent tears were falling non-stop down his cheeks. I stood behind him and held his head against me. There were no words; we were two broken souls that didn't have a language to express our fear or our sorrow.

For the next two days, our house was silent. Neither of us knew what to say, and even the thought of a conversation brought tears to our eyes.

Charles would escape to long periods of deep sleep, while I was lucky to catch a forty-five-minute nap every now and then.

* * *

We arrived at the hospital at five a.m. for Charles' biopsy. We were still silent, but our confusion, pain, and fear was palpable. The doctor stood by the bed and explained the hour-long procedure.

I bent over, kissed Charles on the cheek, and squeezed his hand as they took him to the operating room. I barely made it to the waiting room before breaking down in tears. I slumped into the nearest seat. I held myself and rocked back and forth. The doctor came in and said Charles tolerated the surgery well. He thought it might be Lymphoma but wouldn't be sure until he got the report on Monday. I asked what Lymphoma was and he explained that it was a blood cancer and he would have more information when we came to his office.

I told him I wouldn't be there on Monday because I was leaving for Atlanta to go to the Winship Cancer Center for my own treatment.

"Wow, that is wonderful. They are one of the best in the world. I am so pleased to hear this. Let me know if you need anything from me. I wish you luck, Mrs. Ross. I promise you, I will do everything I can to help your husband."

I went to the recovery area to gather my groggy, tearful husband. I was praying that he would fall into a deep sleep once we got home, but he was restless.

I made soup, and we tried to eat, but couldn't. We hadn't spoken about what the doctor said nor about the fact that I was leaving in less than twenty-four hours. We were now in an emotional void. I gave him a pain pill and he slept. I finished packing my bag, fell on the floor and prayed, and that's where I woke the next morning.

* * *

As I drove to the airport, I pulled over twice. The first time because I was crying and became unsteady behind the wheel. I waited a few

22

minutes, drove a few more miles, and pulled over to vomit. Charles sat in the car and stared ahead. He was in shock, still under the influence of the anesthesia and pain pills.

Once in the airport, I took a seat in the atrium. Charles feebly walked toward the area where Regenia would arrive.

She looked tired but ready to do whatever was required. Her presence was comforting because I knew she loved us and that she was strong and purposeful. Regina was the first of many angels that would be there for us. I could leave with a clear conscience.

I thanked and hugged her. I turned to Charles; it was impossible for us to look at each other without tears, we held each other until I had to walk toward my gate to the unknown in Atlanta.

I found my seat on the plane and looked out the window at the natural beauty of Phoenix. I saw Camelback Mountain in the distance; it does look like a camel with its big hump in the middle, then its long-extended neck and another smaller hump that looks like its head. There is also another rock formation on top of it called the "praying monk" that resembled a man in a long robe at prayer.

We hiked the mountain many times. I was never able to make the summit.

The view from the halfway point was spectacular, but Charles said the panoramic views from the top were breathtaking.

As my plane took off and we passed the mountain, I wondered if either of us would ever see it, much less climb it, ever again. I wondered if there was some truth to the folklore of the "Praying Monk," and if there was, I hoped he was praying for us.

23

Shortly after take-off, I fell asleep. Through my haze, I heard the steward ask, "Ma'am, what will you have to drink?"

As I woke, my hand brushed against my neck. I felt the swelling beneath my ear, which had grown considerably in the last week. My heart skipped a beat, and the words I was going to speak tangled in my throat. I shook my head, and he moved down the aisle.

I laid my head against the window and let the tears trickle down the side of my face and into my ears until I fell asleep. When I woke, the captain was requesting that all passengers fasten their seatbelts for the final descent into Hartsfield-Jackson Airport in Atlanta. The four hours of rest I had on the flight was the most I had at one time in the last two weeks and the most I would get at one time for a while.

* * *

The Atlanta airport is a challenge for the seasoned traveler, the healthy traveler, the domestic or foreign traveler and the young single traveler. It is more difficult for the elderly and physically challenged to navigate. It is a mental, spatial, and physical obstacle course.

I am a seasoned traveler but, my emotional state was handicapping my ability to find my way to the train. I walked around the concourse holding my carry-on for a while before I found my voice to ask for help. A young man showed me where the train was and told me when to get off.

Amid all the emotions of the last few weeks, I had a new feeling; I felt "old." I was looking forward to my fifty-seventh birthday in August, and before this diagnosis, I thought I was in good health. Other than this lump on my neck and a few extra pounds, I didn't think of fifty-six as old. But at that very moment, old was what came to mind.

When I got to the final terminal, I scanned the large crowd, looking for Brooke. When I saw her, I let out a whimper to keep from bawling. I untangled myself from the crowd and grabbed her hand. We couldn't unload our emotions in the middle of the airport, so she grabbed my suitcase from the carousel and we headed to the car.

Once we were outside, I immediately felt the temperature difference between Phoenix and Atlanta. It was cool, and the ground was wet. In a few hours, I traveled from one version of extreme weather to another. It felt exactly like my life at that moment. In a few days, my life went from one extreme to another.

Brooke spoke first, "How are you, Mommy? And how is Papa Charles?"

"Neither of us are good. We are both in a very dark place. I'm fighting to be strong but it's getting harder every minute," I said, my voice trembling.

Brooke's husband, Stevie, appeared at my side. He moved fast and quietly, like a ninja.

His competitive practice of Muay Thai kept him in pique condition, and at six feet and one hundred and seventy pounds he was agile and quick. Before I knew it, he grabbed my bag put it in the trunk and kissed my cheek. With all that action, he hadn't said a word.

My son-in-law and I have always enjoyed a special relationship. There were no mean mother-in-law jokes, no critical comments of how "my daughter could have done so much better." There has only been love and respect.

He lost his mother to breast cancer when he was a teenager and was raised by family members after her passing. She left Jamaica and came to America to work for a wealthy family in New York. Through her hard work and help from her employer, she brought her husband, Stevie, and her young daughters to America. She established a life for them, and her smart, handsome Stevie was the cornerstone of her accomplishments.

"Are you hungry, Mommy? We are starving, and there is nothing ready to eat at the house," Brooke asked.

I didn't have an appetite, but I said yes as I shrank into the backseat of the car. I felt tiny and childlike. I wanted to blurt out "take me to your house right now so you can look at me and tell me everything is going to be alright!"

Instead, I slumped over so low that I could barely see out of the window.

After a quick dinner, we headed to their house. When we arrived, it was almost ten. My granddaughter, Bria, was in bed. I wanted to see her and give her a hug, but that would have to wait.

The guest bedroom was on the first floor and Stevie, with his nimble moves, put my bags in the room and said goodnight. Brooke and I were alone with the lights turned down. I looked at her and recognized that, despite her calm demeanor, her quiet smile, her metered voice, her self-restraint, the one thing she couldn't control when she was afraid was the size of her eyes. They were like two small moons.

As we sat on the couch, she went into business mode.

"Monday we'll go to the hospital and fill out paperwork and maybe meet a few people, then Tuesday I've scheduled an appointment with the First Lady of my church to counsel you and to pray. Do you want to go to church with us in the morning for the eleven o'clock service?"

I reached over and turned the lamp up so the light would shine on our faces. I moved my shoulder-length hair back.

"Look at it." I said, gesturing to the swollen knot behind my ear.

She glanced at it, "Does it hurt?"

"No, it doesn't. I don't feel a thing unless I touch it. No pain, no ache, no heaviness. It's there and has gotten bigger in the last ten days." I felt the tears starting to rise.

"We will get started on this first thing Monday, I promise you, Mommy, you will get the best of care. Stevie and I will do all we can. I talked to Staci about what I know so far, and she is a bundle of tears and nerves. I texted her that you were here now but it's late, and we can talk tomorrow."

We moved to hug each other, and I felt her heartbeat against mine. It reminded me of when she was my little girl and was scared, when I would let her know that everything was going to be okay and that I would be there with her. Now, the roles were reversed.

I listened as Brooke slowly climbed the long staircase. At about the sixth stair, I heard her trying to stifle a cry, but she was unable to contain it. It came out as a thick sob. I sat in my room. The Ninja came swiftly and helped her to their bedroom.

I called Regenia to let her know I was at Brooke's. She said that when they left the airport, they stopped at one of Charles' favorite Mexican restaurants and ate like ravenous wolves. The food was comforting, and Charles relaxed a little. I was glad to hear that he had an appetite.

Sunday morning, I was jet-lagged and feeling the three-hour time difference. At about eight o'clock, I heard someone moving around in the kitchen. It was Bria. She was fixing a bowl of cereal. Before I could take a step into the kitchen, I was almost knocked off my feet by my grand-dog, Kingston. He was jumping and whipping me with his tail.

"Good morning, Mema. Stop it, Kingston!" Bria said.

I hugged her tight and noticed how big she had gotten since I saw her six months earlier, when she celebrated her eleventh birthday with my father at his eighty-fifth birthday party in Cincinnati, Ohio.

I didn't know how much Bria knew about why I was there, so I kept the conversation about school, her soccer team, and the latest songs.

"Where is Papa Charles? How come he didn't come with you?"

"He's still in Arizona. He wanted to come but couldn't."

"Oh, that's right. He must run the restaurant. I wish I were in Arizona. I like working in the restaurant and getting tips when I'm there."

That didn't seem like so long ago, but now we were here, and she was asking me if I wanted her to make me some pancakes.

"No thanks, I'm still full from dinner last night." Bria ran upstairs to get ready for church with Kingston at her heels, and I went back to the guest room.

A few moments later, Brooke knocked on the door and came in looking so beautiful. There was a tiny smile on her face, which was comforting, but again her eyes were big, and they had small dark circles beneath them.

"Good morning, Mommy. Do you want to go to church with us?"

"No, not today. I need to rest and sit still for a moment."

"Okay, we'll put Kingston in Bria's room so that he won't disturb you and we'll be back later. There is food if you want something, and I have a few different coffees you might like."

Before she shut the door, I heard Stevie say, "Good morning, Mommy," and then poof, he was gone.

Once they left, I made myself a nice cup of hot coffee. Though I had on a flannel robe, I was cold.

I opened the back door and looked at the lush green woods. The tall pine trees took the place of the tall palm trees, the bushes were substitutes for the cactus, and the soft green grass replaced the hard-multi-colored rock lawns that I was used to.

I was enjoying the beauty of my surroundings, but my head was reeling from the many changes. I went upstairs and brought Kingston down. For a big, pink-nosed pit bull who was only nine months old, he was very strong and playful. I loved his rust brown color and his one floppy ear.

They were trying to train him, but the success was limited to him going to the door when he needed to go for a walk. He still chewed shoes, or whatever was available. Kingston jumped on the couch and would turn his belly up looking for a long rub from anyone willing to give it. He was comforting; I tried to watch television and he came and laid on my feet and kept them warm.

I wrapped myself in a blanket and turned on the television; I discovered that the news made me uncomfortable. Every station featured shootings, car accidents, a house fire, domestic violence, and war.

I couldn't take it. I found the Animal Planet Channel and listened to Kingston bark every time they showed a cat or dog.

Being with him and watching his reactions made me relax. It was easy because I didn't have to talk or think. With him warming my feet, I started getting bored of the meerkats, and I fell asleep.

Brooke returned from church with the news that my name was on the prayer list. I put on one of Brooke's jackets and went with Bria to walk the dog. Once we turned the corner, she asked me what was wrong. I didn't know what to tell her other than the truth.

"I have cancer, and I came here to go to the hospital that your Mom works at for treatment."

"My other grandma died from cancer. I don't want you to die."

"Baby, I don't want to die either, which is why I am here. The best doctors and the best hospital are right here. I'm going to fight, and they are going to help me."

"I am going to help you too, Mema."

We both smiled as we struggled to hold on to Kingston's leash as he pulled away to chase a squirrel.

30

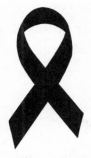

OPERATION
GET MOMMY WELL

Monday morning arrived, and we were on our way to the cancer center. Brooke said she named this challenge: "Operation Get Mommy Well!" She said that for the six years she worked in the cancer field, she was grateful that no one in our immediate family was touched by this disease. Now that I was here, she was going to use everything she learned and every professional contact she knew to "Get Mommy Well!"

I started to feel hopeful and less despondent because she was putting the most important things together: prayer and action.

When we drove into the parking lot, I was surprised at the size of the Winship Cancer Center. I wasn't intimidated, rather, I was impressed. A few people greeted Brooke by name. They asked why she was there, and she replied, "I'm here with my Mom."

A staff member said, "Well Mom, don't worry. You're in a good place and if you need anything, Brooke knows how to reach us."

As we moved through the process of paperwork and scheduling the various tests, my phone rang. It was Regenia I could hear Charles wailing in the background.

"Why? Why me?"

My heart sank into my stomach.

"Bari, we left the doctor's office, and Charles' diagnosis is Acute Lymphoblastic Leukemia. We are on our way to see an oncologist that the doctor recommended, but Charles is inconsolable and won't stop crying."

Regenia is strong, but it was obvious from her panting and the alarm in her voice that this was more than she expected.

"Let me talk to him," I implored.

I could tell Regina had given the phone to Charles because the sound of his cries grew louder in my ear.

"Honey, please stop crying. Listen to me... I love you and we are going to get through this... Do you hear me?"

His words were unintelligible, but I could see his tears pouring through the phone. I couldn't handle it. I asked him to give the phone back to Regenia. I asked her to let me talk to Brooke and to call us once they met with the oncologist.

I looked at Brooke who heard part of the conversation and was anxious to hear the details.

"Charles has Acute Lymphoblastic Leukemia. They are on their way to see an oncologist."

Her head dropped,

"No, Mommy. That's not possible. Both of you can't be this sick with two different cancers at the same time. No, No, No!"

I was now in free-fall. I was no longer trying to keep myself together. I was no longer trying to be strong. I shut down all feelings and became a robot. I decided to move forward like a robot: I will fill the papers out. I will write down appointments. I will walk with one foot in front of the other, and I will remind myself to breathe. I will feel nothing.

When Regenia called after Charles' appointment with the oncologist, I handed the phone to Brooke. She repeated what Regenia was saying.

"The doctor wants to put Charles in the hospital today to begin 23 hour a day chemotherapy, what he has is treatable and has a thirty-five percent cure rate in men his age. The treatment time is about a year and is very intense with lots of hospitalization and various procedures and anticipated setbacks. I explained to the doctor that Bari is in Atlanta for her treatment and that there is no one out here for Charles. I have to leave on Saturday."

Brooke put her on hold. In minutes, she told Regenia to have the oncologist make a peer-to-peer call with another doctor at Winship. I listened but since I willed myself to quit feeling, I didn't ask any questions.

* * *

We went to lunch and Brooke ordered a soup and salad combination.

I passed on the food.

"Mommy, you have to eat, you are going to need strength to get through your treatment. 'Operation Get Mommy Well!' requires all of us to do our part."

I got a small bowl of soup and forced it down to my stomach where my heart had taken up residence.

Brooke received a call from the doctor she worked for who spoke to the oncologist in Phoenix. She held the phone so that I could hear him.

"Make arrangements to get your Dad out here as soon as possible. They need to be together to get through this. It must happen soon. He's in pretty bad shape."

Brooke hung up the phone and breathed a sigh of relief then remembered she had to discuss all of this with her husband. Taking care of two extremely sick people with different needs at the same time was a daunting task.

Brooke called Regenia back. We could still hear Charles in the background crying. I wished that I could ask him to shut down and go robotic like me—not feel anything, but I couldn't. Regenia said she could take Charles back with her to Virginia and have him treated there. She, her husband, and his other sisters could support him. But he was wailing. She felt he needed me, and I needed him. Brooke told her that was what her doctor said.

Charles asked to speak to me, and when Brooke handed me the phone, I said, "Honey, Brooke is working on something to have us together for treatment in Atlanta. Please call Reverend Perry."

34

Reverend Perry was my pastor before I met Charles and he married us. Charles loved and respected him, and I knew the Reverend would be of some comfort to him.

He said that he felt a little better hearing there was a plan. We were in a state of shock. I didn't ask myself what else could go wrong because since I had turned into a robot, it wouldn't matter.

By the time we arrived back to Brooke's house, I was numb all over. I headed straight for the guest room and sat on the bed.

Now that I had more information on my situation and a diagnosis for Charles, I decided I needed to talk to my younger daughter, Staci, and bring her into what was now, "Operation Get Mommy Well… and Papa Charles too!"

I wasn't sure what she knew, but I know that she and Brooke were very close and shared everything with each other—no holds barred. So, I wasn't surprised that when she answered the phone, she was already crying.

"I know you already talked to Brooke and may be up to date about all the unbelievable things that are taking place with Mr. Charles and me, but I want you to know that we are going to fight. Right now, what we need is prayer."

"But Mommy, what happened and why?" she cried.

"Baby, I don't know, and we don't have time to figure those things out. We have to get treatment and help; there is no way Brooke and her family are going to be able to handle all of this."

"Mommy, I am already worried. She is trying to be strong, and I feel guilty that I am up here in Washington, D.C. "

"Don't feel guilty about anything. Give us a few more days, and we will let you know when to come down and what you can do. I love you, and I promise you, as I have everyone else, we are going to fight."

I laid down on the bed and realized I was teary and that I had slipped out of robot mode.

Brooke came in to tell me Stevie said a wholehearted yes to Charles coming to Atlanta. We called Regenia and told here to start working on getting Charles to Atlanta.

Needing spiritual guidance after the traumatic events of the day, Brooke and I went to church to visit with her First Lady. When we entered her office, I was surprised at how young she was. She had such a soft demeanor and the most beautiful eyes. When she spoke her self-confidence and spiritual maturity were on display.

"My counsel to you is that you take authority over this like you have every other problem you've faced up to now. Pray for God's wisdom and grace and keep fighting. Cancer can be defeated."

She, Brooke, and I held hands, and she said a fervent prayer over me for healing, and Brooke for strength in caregiving.

* * *

Regenia was making moves to shut down the remnants of our life in Phoenix. She asked the staff to meet them at the restaurant. They got there before the employees, and Charles broke down, saying that he didn't want to lose the restaurant.

Regenia told him, "If you want a chance at regaining your health and being with Bari, after the meeting you have five minutes to say goodbye to this place and walk away."

Charles needed to make a reservation but didn't have enough money for airfare. He told me he was ashamed to ask Regenia for the money. I suggested he call my friend, Marion, and explain to her what was happening. She offered her American Express Card number and told him to get whatever he needed. Now he was set to come to Atlanta. When I spoke to Regenia, she sounded exhausted but relieved that her assignment was coming to an end.

* * *

Our dear friend and neighbor, Bev, took Regenia and Charles to the airport. When Bev saw how weak and sick Charles was, she helped Regenia get him to the car. When they made it through security, Regenia walked Charles to his gate and then hurried to her flight. Later, Regenia would tell us when she got to her connecting flight in Charlotte, she called her husband and broke down in a puddle of tears.

Four hours later, Stevie and I were at the airport waiting for Charles to make his way through the maze. When I spotted him, I was shocked at how pale and weak he looked. Stevie made his Ninja move over the rope to grab Charles because his legs were folding under him. I grabbed his bag and he sat down on the bench while we waited for Stevie to get the car.

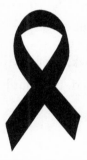

THE WINNING SHIP

We were dealing with what I called "The Fraternal Twin Cancers." Born at the same time but vastly different.

After his flight from Phoenix to Atlanta, Charles was nauseous all night. The next morning, Brooke took him to the emergency room. I had a series of tests scheduled and she was running between areas of the hospital to check on each of us. It seemed impossible, but she managed to pull it off. While I was having a CT Scan, Brooke went to see Charles. When the scan was complete, I went to have an EKG, blood tests, and an x-ray. We went to see Charles. The doctor said he had a severe gastro-intestinal virus and they admitted him to the hospital.

Charles was in isolation. We had to put on a paper gown, a mask, and gloves before we could go into his room. He had several IVs. But he seemed relieved; no crying or hysterics.

When we got home, Stevie and Bria wanted to know why Charles wasn't with us. After Brooke told them he was hospitalized, Bria slipped out of the room with her head down, and Stevie grabbed Kingston and went for a walk. Brooke ordered Chinese food for dinner. We ate in silence and retired to our separate places to try to make sense of the day's events.

Once I was alone in the dark, I asked myself the one question that Charles, Bria, and Staci asked, but that had not been at the forefront of my thinking:

WHY?

Why me, why Charles, why us, why now, why did we lose everything, why are we burdening Brooke and her family, why are we in Atlanta, why is water wet, why is the sky blue?

Then I touched my neck, and all the whys disappeared and were replaced with how? How do I get rid of this lump that is now the size of a ping-pong ball, how does Charles get rid of cancer in his bloodstream, how do we get better and get out of Brooke's home and back into our own?

The how seemed more plausible than the why, so I decided to take authority over the HOW.

* * *

Staci called and said she was coming to Atlanta. She wanted to be with me when the doctors prescribed my treatment.

I was glad Staci was coming. Brooke needed to get back to work and her family, and I needed to see and talk to my Staci.

Brooke prepared Staci for the size of the lump on my neck.

Staci said, "Mom you look the same as you did in February except for the lump. You don't look sick."

"I know. I don't feel sick either, but the doctors here have produced the same diagnosis as the Phoenix doctor. When you and I go to Winship on Monday, we are going to meet my team of doctors. Charles has one doctor who is a Hematologist/Oncologist that treats blood cancers. I have three doctors."

She asked about Charles.

"The stomach virus is still raging, and his immune system has nothing to fight with, but he has calmed. He is looking forward to his daughter and granddaughter coming to visit him next week." I told Staci.

She nodded and said, "I want to be sure to visit him while I'm here."

Staci left my room and I could hear her and Brooke talking in whispers late into the night, like they did when they shared a room as kids.

The next day, we hurried to the hospital to visit with Charles before going to my appointments. Staci saw the sign on the door that said "Isolation." She was alarmed, so I explained to her that we needed to put on all the items in the bin outside his room before entering.

Charles was asleep. The machines were making whirring sounds as they pumped out information and pumped in medication.

I didn't want to disturb him, but our time was short, so I softly called him. He woke up and was surprised to see Staci. He was able to tolerate Ensure, Jell-O, and popsicles, and was hoping to move up to soup and graham crackers.

41

We stayed until Charles began to get sleepy again, then rushed across campus to my appointments.

The first doctor was the ENT surgeon. His specialty was Head and Neck Cancers, which cover the esophagus to the nose.

"I will always be direct with you and never sugarcoat anything," he reassured me.

He looked at the scans and tests but had to wait until he did a pan endoscopy and a tissue biopsy before telling us the stage.

Staci and I spoke at the same time, "What's a pan endoscopy?"

He explained that it is a tiny camera attached to a long tube that takes a panoramic view of the area in the throat and lungs, looking for the primary site of the cancer and how far it may have spread. Once he finds it, there is a tiny set of scissors attached that will cut a piece of the tissue for a biopsy.

This was a plan, a how, a step to solving the problem. He worked very closely with the other doctors I was going to see, but he was the captain of the ship and all decisions of treatment would rest with him. When we arrived to see the Radiologist-Oncologist, I was feeling positive. He had a very different demeanor than the surgeon. When he came into the room, he asked if it was okay to hug me and I said yes. I felt comforted and human by that simple offer. He explained the role of radiation in my treatment to shrink the tumor and kill as much of the cancer cells as possible. The radiation would be used in combination with chemotherapy.

The battle with head and neck cancer was a "real slog," but he was confident that I would make it through. Everything he said made sense but what struck me was the word "tumor." I had been referring to it as swelling, a lump, or a knot.

He used a marker to place dots on the tumor. He walked us to the room where the radiation machine sat. I was shocked at the size. It reminded me of a tunnel. It was long and narrow with what looked like lights. I looked around the room and saw what appeared to be yellow Star Wars masks.

"What are those?" I asked.

"We are going to make a mold of your head and neck today and make one for you to wear when you come for your radiation treatments," he replied.

"It will ensure that you keep your head still and that the radiation is directed precisely to those dots."

Staci went to the waiting room while the technician began making my mold. When I came out, she was on the phone with Brooke and hung up when she saw me. We had one more doctor to see.

I looked down at the schedule and saw that they were kind enough to leave us some time for lunch before the last appointment. We went to the cafeteria in the hospital and had a light meal.

"Mommy, what do you think about the appointments this morning?"

"I was a bit overwhelmed by the information, but I felt good because they seemed to have a three-pronged plan to attack the tumor. I know

I didn't ask a lot of questions. I will come back with a list of things to fill in the blanks."

The medical oncologist explained to us the chemotherapy plan. Until I met him, I thought chemo was as generic for cancer as aspirin is for a headache. He was very courteous, professional, and fastidious.

He explained that the cancer was extremely aggressive, so that the treatment would be more aggressive. The chemo he was prescribing was platinum-based and had a significant rate of success in head and neck cancers.

The downside was that I would be very sick and unable to eat during the seven weeks of radiation and chemotherapy treatment and for a few months after. As if that weren't scary enough, the doctor prescribed a feeding tube so that I could get enough liquid nutrition, like Ensure, to sustain me until I could eat again.

Staci was feverishly taking notes; she wouldn't look at me. I saw a tear sneak down her cheek. I had a thousand questions, but I slipped into robot mode. The doctor noticed my change in demeanor.

"I know it's a lot, but we're are using all the artillery we've got to give you a fighting chance."

He shook my hand, nodded to Staci, and left. His Physician's Assistant came in the door right behind him and gave me the appointment to have the feeding tube inserted. She said the nutritionist and swallowing therapist would contact me with appointments as well.

* * *

We picked up Brooke from work. I sat in the backseat as Staci recounted each appointment. Brooke read all the notes and understood the cancer language that was foreign to us. She assured us that it was a great plan for "Operation Get Mommy Well" and that my doctors were the absolute best for my cancer. It was everything I had prayed for regarding a plan, so I couldn't figure out why I was concerned about the feeding tube.

Once we got to Brooke's house, I went to my room to collect my thoughts. I wasn't sad, but I needed to process the information so that I could ask questions, and since I didn't yet speak the language of cancer, I was frustrated.

I Googled all the words and procedures. I hoped that I had the correct spellings because for many of them, I was guessing or spelling phonetically. It turned out not to be a good idea. The websites I visited either weren't much help or were very frightening. I stopped reading. I needed encouragement, and I couldn't find it in WebMD or Wikipedia.

I called Charles. He sounded much better and more relaxed than he had in months. It made me feel a little lighter knowing that he was getting better from the stomach virus and that tomorrow his doctor would go over the plans to attack the Leukemia.

* * *

When Staci and I walked into Charles' room a few days later, he was sitting up eating a light breakfast. He was still attached to the IV, but there were fewer bags on the pole. His mood had improved, and he was making jokes about how impossible it was to rest in the hospital.

45

"Every thirty minutes someone is coming in the room, waking me up. Sometimes it's the nurse to check my medicine, and then the techs to check my blood pressure and temperature, then someone to take a blood sample, then another person comes to clean the room, then they come to bring food. I need to get out of here to get some sleep."

As he finished, the doctor came in the room.

She was a petite woman with a very efficient manner. She was courteous to Staci and me, but she was laser-focused on Charles. She explained that she specialized solely in cancers of the blood and their test confirmed that Charles had Acute Lymphoblastic Leukemia, or ALL.

She began writing on the whiteboard. Staci was furiously capturing every word like a court reporter. I was lost in the language, but I did pick up the fact that his leukemia was rare in adults, was typically diagnosed in young children, and that "acute" meant that the disease could progress quickly if not treated. It would probably be fatal if left untreated a few months.

She drew pictures of blood cells and bone marrow.

She was taking her time to educate us in simplistic terms, but it was too much for me to grasp. I sat and watched Charles to see his reaction to what the doctor was saying, and I would gauge my response accordingly. He was nodding and saying okay. I thought that was strange and then I remembered he might have heard some of this with the doctor in Phoenix.

He asked her how he got this disease and she said that it was indeterminate; her goal was to get him into remission. She told him the primary treatment was an aggressive chemotherapy protocol. He would be hospitalized and given chemotherapy twenty-three and a half hours a day for six weeks. He would have minor surgery to implant a "port or catheter" into his chest to deliver the medicine into his system.

Because of the amount and duration of treatment, it could not be done through his arm. Staci asked about radiation and surgery, and she said neither of those are used. Should the chemotherapy not work, there may be a need for a bone marrow transplant, but she wanted to give the chemo a chance. The survival rate for sixty+-year-old men with this disease was about 35%, but she would use everything available to help him.

Charles blurted out, "My wife has cancer too, and she is starting treatment here soon."

The doctor turned around, and I saw the naked surprise on her face, "May I ask what you have, Mrs. Ross?"

I couldn't speak. Staci explained to her who my doctors were and my diagnosis.

She blinked hard and stood still for a few seconds. "I am sorry. I've never heard of a couple having two aggressive cancers at the same time. Winship is one of the best cancer centers in the world, and each of you will get leading-edge treatment here."

She slowly erased the pictures from the whiteboard. She wrote her name and number in large letters on the corner of the board and told Charles to call her if he had any questions.

Staci asked Charles how he felt about what the doctor said.

"I have surrendered. I will do everything they say... whatever it is, whenever they say to do it. I don't have any questions because I don't know what to ask. I want to survive."

Staci let a slight smile curl at the corners of her mouth and repeated: surrender.

She stepped out to call Brooke and give us some time alone. I updated Charles on what my doctors said about my treatment plan. He couldn't imagine what they were proposing but encouraged me to surrender and not to try to out-think the doctors. I felt conflicted because I was thinking that I needed to take "authority" of the situation, not understanding how surrendering could accomplish that.

As I was leaving, a parade of nurses, techs and housekeeping started arriving in his room. I rubbed his cheek and slid out the door past the incoming lunch cart.

Staci wanted a burger from the Vortex restaurant, so we headed there for lunch. When we pulled up, I was taken aback; the doorway was a huge screaming white skull. Staci is a "foodie" and always treats me to unusual and exciting places to eat. There were skulls everywhere in the décor and on the menu.

"This food must be to die for," I joked.

At first, I thought it was funny, but dying was the last thing I wanted to think about.

* * *

When Staci was in Phoenix a few months before, she took us to a chic pizza restaurant in Phoenix that I didn't know existed nor did I care, because every night there was a minimum two-hour wait for a table, and they didn't take reservations. But we waited so she could tell her other "foodie friends" that she had been there.

"What is going on with you? Tell me something good," I said as I looked over the menu.

She had met a new guy. As she spoke, her eyes sparkled, and her face beamed.

Staci ordered "The Plain Ol' Original Vortex Burger" with fries, and I ordered the "Zombie Apocalypse."

I couldn't eat more than a few bites as she told me about her new job and the new man in her life. It felt good to have one of our girl talks. I enjoyed the time with her, sitting in the middle of a skull being served by a waitress in full Goth costume and makeup. When I looked at this place, maybe the two-hour wait for the gourmet pizza hadn't been so bad.

After lunch, Staci and I went to meet Brooke at her house. Brooke confirmed that Charles' doctor was one of the best in the field of blood cancers. Not only did she see patients, but she was involved in teaching, research, and clinical trials. Brooke was glad to hear that Charles had surrendered and said that would make his treatment go better. I listened to the "hint, hint Mommy" in her voice and saw it in Staci's eyes. Bria came downstairs and joined us, and the four of us watched the movie "The Color Purple," with each of us one picking a character and speaking their lines. Kingston came and laid on my feet, and I felt good being in the middle of the love and care from my girls.

***

My pan endoscopy was on Monday morning. Brooke was going to be there with me. Staci left; she would be back in two weeks and promised to come often. She was as concerned about Brooke as she was about Charles and me. I have always loved their sister relationship and have made it a point to stay out of "sister stuff." When they would have disagreements growing up, and one or the other would ask me to intervene, I would always say "sorry, I am the mother, and I don't do 'sister stuff.' That's for the two of you to work out." Their love and care for each other were shining through, and I took the time to bask in the glow.

Charles' daughter, granddaughter, and ex-wife came to Atlanta to visit him. When they walked into the hospital room and saw him attached to the IVs and saw his depleted appearance, they cried.

I had been with Brooke for three weeks. I felt like a sponge. I reached out to my sister, Traci. She was shocked and had no idea that I left Phoenix and when I told her about Charles, I could hear the breath escape her chest. I wasn't trying to hide, but I knew people would have lots of questions for which I had no answers, and some would rush to horrific conclusions without information.

I trusted that she would honor my request not to share our situation with anyone. I asked her to send me money to help with my expenses. Two days later when it arrived in the mail, it felt like a million dollars; each act of kindness felt like a winning lottery ticket.

***

It was time for my first of many surgeries; this was the surgery the ENT would use to determine the stage of the tumor.

"How is the 'stage' assessed?" I asked.

He handed me the information.

I tried to follow the discussion, but it was like alphabet soup. I thought Brooke might be able to explain it to me later.

The doctor said that after the surgery, my throat would be sore for a few days and that there may be light bleeding, but it was nothing to worry about.

I looked at Brooke's eyes to gauge her feelings. She was calm, I exhaled my concerns and inhaled the anesthesia.

The doctor said that he found the primary site of the cancer and it was the size of a nickel and had spread outside of the immediate area. He added that he would have further details for me in two days time and to call for an appointment.

On the way home, the painkiller started to wear off, and my throat and head were hurting. The doctor gave me a prescription for a mild sedative, and we stopped to have it filled. I was tired and grumpy. Brooke dropped it off and took me home. I went to sleep without changing my clothes. Two hours later, I woke up and my throat was on fire, and my head felt like it was jumped on by a small army of toddlers.

Stevie brought me the medication. It was hard to swallow. Once I got it down, I ate a small bowl of chicken broth with some warm tea. I changed clothes, went to sleep, and slept through the night undisturbed by pain, by dreams, and by possibilities. Once my head was clearer, I talked to Brooke about the staging. She said she and Staci discussed it and based on what they read, they thought it was stage 2 or 3. It sounded reasonable and hopeful to me.

I called Charles to tell him what stage we thought my cancer was in, but it was hard for him to relate because leukemia is not 'staged' as cancers that have solid tumors. He said his niece, Angie, who lived in the area, came by to visit him and brought fresh fruit. He also heard from his nephew, DeVance, and was feeling the love of his extended family. He called his son and shared his diagnosis with him. His son said he would send money and hoped to visit him. I was glad that he was being comforted by others since I was surrounded by Brooke, Stevie, Bria, and Kingston.

My throat was still achy. I gargled with warm saltwater, took a pain pill, and went to bed. I was anxious, but I knew I had to face the "big reveal" the next day, and each step after that would be a march uphill in "Operation Get Mommy Well."

The next morning as we stepped out of the elevator, Charles was walking towards us holding on to the pole with two or three bags hanging like laundry. He was smiling, and he seemed proud to be out of bed and moving. His infection was gone; he could leave his room. His doctor prescribed ten laps around the floor. Walking made him feel good. I said I would do a lap and give him a few steps head start since I didn't have to pull a pole of medications. We laughed and decided to hold hands and walk at the same pace.

***

We arrived at my appointment and the nurse took us to an area that was further away from the previous rooms. I felt a sense of déjà vu when I walked in and noticed there was box of Kleenex on the table.

I looked at Brooke and she said, "Mommy, don't read anything into it. This is an information session, not an exam."

The Captain walked in, shook our hands, and sat down heavily in the chair.

"Mrs. Ross, you know I told you I don't sugar coat the facts. I have some news that is hard for me to say and I'm sure will be harder for you to hear."

I investigated his pale blue eyes for anything other than what his mouth was saying. I was looking for sadness, hope, compassion, sympathy, peace, optimism but before I could find any of those my ears, I heard the words STAGE 4B.

I turned my head like a boxer when he receives a knockout punch. I looked at Brooke as I fell into the abyss and her face was down writing frantically, but I could see her large moon eyes.

I didn't faint, but I took an eight-count waiting for the blood and air to reach my brain. The doctor said I would begin radiation and chemo within the next week and that, despite my resistance, they couldn't treat me unless I agreed to a feeding tube, which should be in place the next two days. I was scheduled to begin radiation and chemotherapy on the same day in exactly one week.

He gave Brooke a packet of information, looked at me and said, "Our team is committed to you. It is a plus that you are in excellent health with no other issues except this cancer and that will go a long way in helping your fight. I know it's not what you wanted to hear, but that's where we are."

I did not speak as he left the room.

Brooke and I sat in silence for a while. Without a word, she helped me out of the chair. Once I gained my balance, we walked down the long hallway, past all the rooms where people were undergoing tests; they would be sitting where I was in a few days to get 'staged.'

I don't remember getting in the car or the drive home. We floated home on a dark cloud that carried us over the crazy Atlanta rush hour traffic without hearing any horns blow, without seeing the homeless men begging for money on the entrance to the highway, without changing lanes or stopping for lights. We floated our way through the garage door without using the remote and through the door without using the key. We had to float because our legs could not hold us up.

The dark cloud landed me softly in my bed. The dark cloud dropped Brooke on the couch in the living room, holding her cell phone, reporting and comforting Staci's tears and screams from five hundred miles away. The dark cloud sent my confused Bria running up to her room again but without Kingston following her. The dark cloud handicapped the Ninja moves of Stevie, so when he grabbed his wife it was in slow motion. They moved up the stairs holding on to the railing and each other like an elderly arthritic couple, unlike like the spry newlyweds they were. The dark cloud floated Kingston to lay outside the door of my room whimpering softly, as if he also knew what STAGE 4B meant.

54

PRIMARY TUMOR

TX Primary tumor cannot be assessed

T0 No evidence of primary tumor

Tis Carcinoma in situ

T1 Tumor 2 cm or less in greatest dimension

T2 Tumor more than 2 cm but not more than 4 cm in greatest dimension

T3 Tumor more than 4 cm in greatest dimension or extension to lingual surface of epiglottis

T4a Moderately advanced local disease

T4b Very advanced local disease

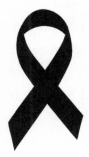

PRACTICAL THINGS

"Bari, as long as the sun rises in the east and sets in the west, you have a new day in which you can move forward," is what my dad always told me.

My dad was the person I always turned to when I faced challenges or failures. He counseled me wisely when I needed it and scolded me when necessary. The one thing he never did was give me bad advice.

With that in mind, when I woke up and looked out the window and saw the sun was rising in the east, I had to decide what I was going to do with the day. Brooke and Stevie were at work, and Bria was at school. When I opened the door, Kingston was in front of it. He jumped up and licked my hand and waited for my reaction. I patted him on the head and he dropped to the floor and offered me his belly. I rubbed it slowly to show him gratitude for protecting me through the night.

I had no appetite, but I made myself eat oatmeal. I sat down and made a list of people I needed to contact now that I knew the extent of Charles' and my own diagnoses. It was heartbreaking because, after

Charles, my eighty-seven-year-old Dad was at the top of the list. His health was starting to deteriorate the last few years as evidenced by a series of falls and getting lost when he drove. My brother, Herman Jr, passed two years before from cancer, and Dad grieved hard for quite a while. As much as I tried, I couldn't bring myself to call him. He thought we were still in Phoenix.

It occurred to me that this required an intervention, and I knew the people to do it. I called Traci, my brother Tim, and his wife, Arlene, on a three-way line and told them the stage and the treatment plan for me. They were shocked. I asked them to go along with Debbie, my best friend since we were twelve years old, who Dad calls his other daughter, to tell him. I ask them to promise that once they told him and saw his reaction to tell me and then I would call him.

Then I called Debbie. When I told her the news, she screamed into the phone, "No, Devil, no. You can't take my sister!"

I asked her to join my sister and brother to tell Dad. Debbie said yes and until that time, she would ask her church to pray for us. I was relieved and felt that Dad and his wife, Mary, were in the best hands and would be surrounded by love and support when they heard the news.

As a practical matter, there were still things I needed to take care of before I began treatment.

I needed to get my haircut. In reading through the material, I found that some chemo and some radiation doses cause hair to fall out. I didn't want the additional trauma of my hair coming out in clumps, a little at a time, so I decided to shave it in advance. Hair was the least of my worries. I also needed to see the dentist before treatment to make sure my teeth and gums were healthy.

Yes, the practical things still had to be managed, so I put on my clothes, grabbed the leash, and took Kingston for a walk because he was sitting impatiently by the door.

I was active; there was nothing about me that said I had late-stage cancer except the large tumor under my right ear.

It was late spring in Atlanta and the weather was perfect. It was sunny, the sky was clear, the wind was light, and the temperature was 75 degrees. I said a silent prayer and thanked God for such a day.

Kingston saw a squirrel and almost dragged me off my feet. I allowed myself to laugh at this silly puppy who thought he could run up the tree after the squirrel.

When I got back to the house, Debbie called to let me know that she spoke to Traci and Tim and they were going to tell Dad on Sunday afternoon.

I still hadn't decided when I was going to tell Charles. There was no easy way, none of this has been easy, but again my heart was rendered in pieces at the thought of bringing him down when he seemed to be stable on an emotional balance beam, and one tiny misstep could send him spiraling downward.

When I called Charles, he was excited that Regenia and Jerry were coming to Atlanta for the weekend. He was looking forward to thanking them and he wanted Regenia to see the progress he'd made. He asked what the doctor said about my biopsy. I told him I thought it best if I explained in person.

"Okay, I'll see you tomorrow."

I laid down for a nap and Kingston took his position. When I woke up, Bria was coming through the door from school.

"Hi, Mema."

She had too much worry on her face for an eleven-year-old.

"Bria, don't worry. Papa Charles and I are going to be fine. It's going to take a while, but we're going to be around a long time. There may be times when we need your help, but if it's too much or interferes with your schoolwork or fun, say so."

She nodded and hugged me. As she started to leave the room, she called out—

"Come, Kingston."

The playful dog ran over to her, licked her hand, then came and sat beside me.

"Wow, Mema, I guess he needs to be with you right now."

I tried to shoo him towards her, but he wouldn't move. I realized that some angels have furry wings.

When Brooke came into my room a little while later, she looked tired.

"Mommy, we were not expecting Stage 4B. You have got to fight with everything you have. We need you to be strong and we also news need you to surrender to the doctors the way Papa Charles did. Staci and

60

I are working on a list of people who can come and help over the next few months, and if you can think of anyone who can help for a few days, a week, or even a few hours a day, let us know. I've been gathering information and forms so that you and Papa Charles can file for Social Security Disability, Medicare, the American Cancer Society and other Social Services; also, there is a program through the hospital to help with medical expenses. I've asked that you be assigned a Social Worker and a Financial Counselor. Staci is coming to be with you for your first week of treatment."

Brooke touched my hand and before the tears could rain down, she left.

It was evident that "Operation Get Mommy Well" had evolved into "Operation Save Mommy's Life," which now needed a different strategy and more troops.

Yes, the practical things must be dealt with, even though I had Stage 4B head and neck cancer and my husband had leukemia.

I could hear Kingston breathing outside of the door. As I drifted off to sleep, I heard my Dad's voice say, "Bari, you moved forward today you can do the same tomorrow."

* * *

Brooke had a friend who offered to cut my hair. I got up early so Stevie could show me how to use the GPS in the car, so that I could get around to do my "practical things."

I had never driven in Atlanta, but Stevie assured me that the talking GPS would lead me to the door of any place I needed to go if I had the address. I would have preferred a map or a printout of turn by turn directions, but I had no choice but to go with the new technology.

I made it to the beautician's house without a problem. When she looked at my long, thick hair, she couldn't imagine why I wanted to shave it all off. I told her why and she reluctantly started cutting it by the handful but couldn't bring herself to shave it bald. She said she would pray for me. I asked her to include my husband in all prayers because he had cancer as well. She put her head in her hands, sat down on her couch and cried.

* * *

With my new haircut, it was now time to go to the hospital to tell Charles the news.

When I got in the car and turned on the GPS, it didn't work. All it kept saying was, "searching for satellite…"

After five minutes, I went back to the beautician's door and asked her if she could help me with directions to the hospital. She said that she could get me back to the highway, but she didn't know how to get to the hospital and that maybe once I started driving, the GPS would kick on. I was trying not to panic, so I remained calm and followed her directions. Once, I made it to the highway, I knew to go north but not where to get off or what to do when I exited.

I pulled over and called Brooke; she wasn't at her desk. I reached Stevie, and he stayed on the phone with me for the thirty-minute drive.

As I pulled into the hospital's parking area, the GPS announced, "you have reached your destination on the left."

62

* * *

When I walked into Charles' room, he gasped, "Honey what happened to your hair!"

Before I could answer, he screamed, "Oh my God, look at your neck!!"

Without my long hair to cover it, the tumor was apparently very noticeable.

I looked in the mirror in his bathroom. It was shocking— my face and head seemed as grotesque as the "House of Mirrors" that make you look distorted. The tumor looked like I was sprouting another head.

Charles stood up from the chair and threw his arm, the one that was not tethered to the IV, around me and held me tightly.

"I still love my wife no matter what."

Without skipping a beat, I told him what the doctor said. At first, he didn't understand what Stage 4B meant because there are no stages in Leukemia, but when I showed him the chart, he slumped back in the chair. The tears came, followed by the air leaving his body.

The nurse suddenly appeared at the door. I hadn't heard the machines going off. She rushed past me and helped Charles back into the bed. She asked me to step out of the room. I heard him crying and trying to explain to her what I told him. A few minutes later, another nurse appeared with a cart. I went to a waiting room down the hall.

I paced in circles feeling guilty and ashamed. After about fifteen minutes, one of the nurses told me they gave him a sedative. I told her since he was calm, I would leave.

When I got to the car, I turned on the GPS and pressed 'Home'. The artificial voice started up. I was grateful.

I felt like I was on the precipice of insanity. How could I feel guilty or responsible for any of this? How could I be ashamed that I, or we, had cancer? I had no answers to either question. I drove home listening to the GPS voice telling me when to turn left or right in 200 feet.

***

The next day, I decided not to go to the hospital. I would wait for Regenia and Jerry to come to Atlanta. I spoke to Charles on the phone, and he was so groggy that I could hardly make out his words.

I filled out the forms that Brooke gave me. I went to see the dentist who was surprised to see my tumor. She was professional and cordial, but her eyes betrayed her training.

I immediately addressed the elephant in the room. Once I told her my diagnosis, she asked if it was discovered in a dental check-up. I said no. She asked if I drank, smoked, chewed tobacco, or did street drugs. I said no to all. She asked if she could bring in one of her associates to see my tumor. I didn't have a problem with her request if what I had could be used as a learning tool. She examined my mouth thoroughly and signed the required papers saying my teeth and gums were perfect.

On the way home, I stopped at Target to look for a dress to wear to church. I had exactly twenty-five dollars and I found a decent summer sheath on sale for $19.99. I didn't care about price, labels, or fabric; I needed to be covered and presentable. I was in and out in less than twenty minutes.

The next morning, Regenia called from a nearby hotel. I wanted to talk to them before our visit with Charles. When they picked me up, they were shaken to see my short hair and the size of the tumor. I told them about the stage of my tumor. My cool, calm, and collected brother-in-law held his breath and turned his head to the side. He'd lost his mother to cancer and he was familiar with the language.

I explained to Regenia that we were going to need family and friends to provide hands-on help with our care over the next few months.

When we got to the hospital, Charles was sitting in the chair having lunch. Regenia told him how much better he looked since she saw him at the airport. He said he felt much better and that he was on a half-hour break from his chemo. Charles asked them if they knew about my diagnosis and if they saw my tumor. They nodded yes. He started tearing up, and Regenia moved fast. She held his hand and told him to look how far he'd come in a few weeks with the treatment he was getting, and the same thing would happen to me.

The nurse walked in and said she needed to start the chemo again and give him some additional medications.

"What other medicines?" I asked.

She looked at Charles, and he said his doctor prescribed anti-anxiety and anti-depression medication. The nurse explained that it was not unusual for patients undergoing cancer treatments to take these medications but given the high level of stress he was under; it was necessary for him.

Regenia, Jerry, and I stepped out of the room. In the few short hours since they arrived in Atlanta, Regenia and Jerry looked worn down from the typhoon of events that was now my everyday existence.

After the nurses started Charles' next round of chemo, we stepped back in the room. Charles was slipping off to sleep. Jerry shook his hand and gave him a "Virginia is for Lovers" t-shirt. Regenia told him the family sent their love and prayers.

Regenia and Jerry drove me home and stopped in to see Brooke's family. Regenia thanked them for stepping up in a big way to take care of us. She promised that she and the rest of the family in Virginia would do whatever was needed to help.

Staci came in later, and I knew Brooke warned her about my appearance. Nevertheless, she couldn't hide her surprise at how pronounced the tumor was. She asked me again if it hurt. Staci was the first family member who asked to touch it and seemed surprised about how hard it was.

"Mommy, you still don't seem sick. I don't understand how you can be up moving around, driving, and going to see Mr. Charles."

I said nothing because I didn't understand it either.

I left them sitting on the couch and headed to my room. Kingston took his place at the door.

The next morning, I got up early and called Charles. He had a good night's sleep and was waiting for his breakfast. I reminded him that I was going to have the operation to insert the feeding tube in two days. I probably wouldn't see him until I began chemo and radiation. I told him that Staci would come by to see him and bring videos and snacks while I was in surgery.

* * *

The next morning, Brooke and I stepped into her church, people were rushing up to her, offering their help and prayers. Brooke was overwhelmed by the outpouring. She introduced me to many of them, but one person stood out because of what she said.

"Hi, I'm Brooke's friend Britta. It is so awesome that God has given you the opportunity to go through this. When you recover you will have a powerful testimony to share with the world."

I was perplexed.

I thought to myself, how is having cancer awesome or an opportunity?

I couldn't dwell on it because the organ music started, and it was time to take a seat.

When we got home, Staci suggested we go out for Sunday Brunch. My "Foodie" daughter wanted to treat us to another new place. We were all in agreement that we needed a treat and this may be my last feast for a while.

* * *

When we arrived at the trendy new restaurant, it was full. I was feeling anxious about how things were progressing with my family, so I stepped away to call Traci. I wanted to find out when they were going to talk to Dad. When I was walking back to my seat, a man was talking to his wife and pointed at my neck. I stopped in my tracks as

67

the flames of shame engulfed me. These random emotions of guilt, embarrassment, and shame were attacking me from all sides, and I had nowhere left to put them. I lowered my eyes and kept walking.

Staci was telling us about her new guy and how supportive and loving he was. She reached into her purse and handed me a box. When I opened it, I saw a beautiful soft, tan, clay angel with wire wings. She said her boyfriend told his uncle in Texas about what was going on and his uncle sent him the angel to give to us. I was grateful for the angel but more thankful that Staci had someone special in her life that she could confide in and that his care for her extended to us. We enjoyed the food and the family time and headed home too full to talk. When I got to my room, I put the angel on the table near my bed.

***

Debbie called, and her voice was shaking. She said when they got there, Daddy and Mary weren't home. Tim suggested they sit at the picnic table in the backyard and wait. They didn't hear the car pull up, but Mary recognized Tim's car and heard their voices and came to the back. She was surprised to see all four of them and showed them to the basement where Dad was getting ready to watch his beloved Cincinnati Reds.

Debbie told me she spoke first, and said "Daddy Herman and Miss Mary, we have something to tell you."

"What is it?" they asked in unison.

Debbie continued, "Bari is in Atlanta with Brooke, and she has cancer."

68

Daddy screamed, "Oh no, not Cootsie," as he fell backward into the stairwell. Tim moved to catch him, and Traci rushed to his side. Mary was in shock, and Arlene was running between them trying to help while blotting her tears.

They were crying and trying to gather themselves, and Debbie knew that her task was only half done. She breathed deeply and told them about Charles. The room exploded with a barrage of questions, moans, tears, wailing, sobs, agony, retching, and then stunned silence. When they were satisfied that Dad and Mary were somewhat stable, they left to go to return to their respective homes to sort out the feelings that engulfed them.

I could vividly picture what took place. I was all cried out. I thanked her. She started to pray and cry and then cry and pray. She was exhausted, but like a real soldier, she completed her mission.

Three hours later, I got a call from Tim. He and Arlene were back at Dad's house. He said that the paramedics left a few minutes before. Dad's blood sugar dropped from the shock. Mary said he was talking to her, and suddenly he started slurring his words and speaking gibberish. She turned to look at him, and he collapsed. She called 911 and then called him. When he got there the EMT's were administering glucose and had Dad on an IV. He started coming around. They asked him if he would go with them to the hospital and he refused. Mary was confident that she could handle him until she could get him to his doctor the next day.

I still couldn't cry. All I could think was that cancer had not only metastasized in my body, but its impact was metastasizing throughout my family.

* * *

The next morning, I was laying in the recovery room with a long plastic tube hanging out of my stomach above my navel. I was afraid to touch it. I couldn't feel it, but it looked foreign. I had no frame of reference, but I had to get used to it because it was now as much a part of me as the cancer that caused it to be there.

Staci returned from visiting Charles and had good news. He would be coming home in two weeks for a ten-day break from his chemo, though he would still have outpatient visits for blood platelets. The nurse came in to show us how to use the feeding tube. Staci tried to follow her directions step by step and was successful after two attempts at getting water into my stomach. The only sensation I felt was cold. The nurse showed her how to clean the area and sent us on our way with a bag of gauze, tape, and large plastic syringes.

On the way home, I told Staci about my Dad's reaction,

"Poor Granddaddy, it must be a lot for him. When are you going to call him?"

"I want to wait until after he sees his doctor, and I will speak to Mary first."

"After you get some rest and Brooke gets home, we are going to put together a chart of caregivers, availability, and appointments for the next two months. I will come down every two weeks, but for the other

70

weeks, Brooke has to have help."

"I have a few names and phone numbers, but I'm not sure how many of those could or would commit to a week."

"I will contact them and create the chart for whatever time people are available. Brooke and Stevie offered that if they were coming from out of town, they could stay in the extra bedroom upstairs that way they could be hands-on for you whenever you need it. Since you are starting treatment in two days, it is imperative that this is complete tonight."

I learned that caregivers are as crucial to the patient as the doctors and the medicines. They are unique angels sent from seventh heaven. They are selfless, generous, and sacrificing beyond measure. They give their time, energy, and resources. Most of all, they are what love looks like.

Each name we suggested fit the description. The list included Debbie, Charles' sisters—Polly and Shirley, two of my longtime friends who lived in the Atlanta area—Lois and Monica, Traci, and of course, Regenia. The other names were put on the bench, but the starting lineup was set. Staci took out a calendar and wrote down the appointments I had for daily radiation for the next seven weeks. She wrote down my bi-weekly chemo treatments and the clinic appointments for Charles when he wasn't in the hospital. It looked like an air traffic control screen with all the comings and goings plotted to intersect at just the right time.

"Operation Save Mommy's Life" was now in full effect, at least on paper. Staci and Brooke seemed calmer and able to look at everything that needed to be done, without feeling they needed to do it all. I looked at the schedule and thanked God for angels whether human, clay, or canine.

The next day was going to take me two places that I never thought I would find myself, in the infusion center for chemo and in a long tube under a mask where a beam would send radiation into my tumor.

I was nervous, but confident that God answered my prayers for a plan to save my life. Even if the plan called for me to walk through the abyss of hell for the next few months. it was a chance to live.

We entered the Radiation Oncology department. The receptionist was friendly and courteous. She showed me how to sign in every day on the computer. It wasn't until I turned the corner of the waiting room that I stared the devastation of head and neck cancer in its ugly face.

I turned to look away from a man with the bottom half of his face missing, though it was covered by what looked like a mini-drape, only to see a woman in her mid-forties with a hole in her face where her nose once resided.

There were several people with severely burned necks. I read in the materials that people who have radiation may get what appears to be a severe sunburn. These seemed more akin to the pictures I've seen of burn victims with layers of skin peeling like onions. There was a young man whose skull looked like it caved in on itself, his mother was explaining to another caregiver that he had brain cancer and that the tumor had been removed surgically along with part of his skull, which would be restored with a prosthetic plate.

Many people sat with their heads down. Others were looking out into space as if the answer to their suffering lay out there. The only noise that many responded to was their name when the tech came to escort them to the treatment area. I could see that Staci was also affected because her head was down like she was writing, but there was nothing on the page.

"Bari Ross," an amiable man named Greg greeted me. He walked over and hooked his arm underneath mine like a true southern gentleman. He winked and told Staci he would have me back in fifteen minutes and instructed her to help herself to the gourmet hospital coffee.

As we headed towards the room, I saw more patients who were missing various parts of their once whole bodies, whether it was a leg, an eye, a breast or a voice— since they were here, it meant they had lost it to cancer.

Greg presented me with my mask and joked,

"Does this look like you?"

I replied it did not.

"Well, when I put it on you. if it fits your face, and I line it up with the dots on your tumor, we'll know whether it's you or not."

The other tech asked me if I was claustrophobic. If I was, the nurse could give me a light sedative.

I didn't want sedation. I wanted to see and hear what was happening.

The tech laid me down and put the mask over my face and fastened it in place to hooks on the table.

I was completely immobilized and was glad to be able to breathe. The technicians left the room, and I heard the machine start with a slow whirr. Greg's voice was coming through a speaker in the room, "Close your eyes, Mrs. Ross. You are going to hear a series of dull buzzes and clicks. Please, under no circumstances should you move. I will let you know when you're done."

I laid there listening to the machine's noises without a thought and waited to hear his voice again.

The other tech came through the door followed by Greg. She moved around the table and freed me from the mask. Greg helped me down from the table and said I had done well. He delivered me back to Staci and said he would see me tomorrow, then he called out the name of his next hopeful patient.

Staci had the schedule for the morning, and she said our next stop was the Infusion Center. This was my first time in the place, and I did not know what to expect. When we got to the waiting room, I was taken aback by the number of people. There were two waiting areas and both were at full capacity. Staci stood in line to complete the paperwork and get my ID bracelet while I went to find seats.

As I looked around, I noticed that the patients in here were different than in radiology-oncology. There was not as much visible disfiguration, but there were malaise and sickness apparent in almost every face, including the faces of the caregivers. I understood from my reading that some cancer patients get chemotherapy and later

74

get radiation but because my cancer was aggressive and advanced, I would be doing both simultaneously. That meant that I would be disfigured and sick at the same time.

When my name was called, the technician showed us to a bay that had one large leather chair that looked like a recliner on steroids and one small metal chair. There was a little personal size TV hanging on a big support bar in front of the recliner. The technician pulled the curtain around the area and brought me a warm blanket.

I looked at Staci and she seemed nervous, but I remained calm as the nurse slid around the drape. She started an IV line in my arm. Staci's head was down as she wrote like a cub reporter for a newspaper. I knew she didn't like needles, so I told her to stand outside of the curtain until the nurse finished.

The pharmacist came to explain the chemo would be very potent and have many side effects. I would be given three doses over the six weeks and each one would take approximately two hours to administer through an IV drip. The side effects may include nausea, tingling in hands and feet, dizziness, dry mouth, and lethargy. I didn't have any questions, and Staci took her court stenographer position and never looked up from her writing.

It took an hour before my bag of chemo arrived. I was surprised at its size. I was expecting it to be a quart, but it looked like less than a pint. Based on its size, I couldn't imagine why it would take two hours or more, but once the chemo started to trickle down the line in individual drops, I understood. Staci said she was going to get lunch and then see Charles. It was also implicit that she was going to call

75

Brooke and make her live report of the morning's events.

I tried to watch the TV but couldn't find anything of interest. I turned it off and then I heard it—people retching and vomiting throughout the area. It was like a chorus, some were low followed by moans, others high followed by heaves, and a few mid-range wails followed by gasping. I prayed that I wouldn't be part of that choir, but it seemed inevitable. I tried to doze off, but the chorus grew louder as more patients entered the bay.

After an hour, I slipped into a nap. When I woke up, Staci was sitting in the small chair looking at a magazine, and the nurse was standing over me checking the IV. For a few seconds, I was confused about where I was, and then I recognized the sounds of gagging and all confusion cleared away. When it was time to go, the nurse told me to drink plenty of liquids. She gave me a box of green emesis "sickness bags" to use if needed. She gave Staci the day's paperwork and the information for the next appointment.

* * *

"Do you feel any different, Mommy?" Staci asked as we sat in the interminable Atlanta traffic in the way hone.

"No, I feel the same… as a matter of fact, I'm hungry. Could we stop somewhere and eat?"

"That's good, I will treat you to whatever you want."

I opted for a good meal of southern soul food with sweet tea. I ate most of it and was proud of myself.

When we got home my mood changed. I was exhausted and wanted to be left alone. I didn't want to talk or listen. Kingston came and sat on my feet and began to whimper. I thought to myself, he's never done that before. Usually, he's a licking, silent sentinel.

I went into the bedroom to lie down, and Brooke came in behind me. She read Staci's notes and wanted to know what I thought about the events of the day. "Everybody there was considerate, and I liked my radiation-oncology tech, he made me laugh."

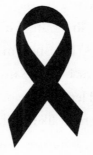

IT'S THE
CANCER, MOMMY

It was about one o'clock at night when it started. I woke up, and my left-hand was tingling. I thought I had fallen asleep on my arm and rolled over to my right side. Within minutes, my right hand started to tingle. I sat up in the bed and decided to get up. Once I tried to stand up and put pressure on my feet, I fell back into the bed. My feet felt like thousands of pins were pricking them. Tears of pain welled in my eyes, and a white lightning bolt went up the back of my neck straight to my brain. I laid there waiting for it to pass. I didn't want to wake up the house, so I laid there. Kingston was stirring by the door, but he didn't bark; he also just laid there.

After about an hour, the pain subsided. I limped into the bathroom. Kingston was at my heels and it looked like he was limping too. As I got ready to sit, my brain sent a strong signal that I would have to choose between sitting or falling to my knees. I dropped to my knees and watched remnants of collard greens, black-eyed peas and yams rushing out of me in tidal waves. I held on to the toilet bowl feeling like I would be swept away if I didn't. When it subsided, I tried to stand up, but the tide came in again. This continued until there was nothing left but clear liquid. I pushed myself up, holding on to the tub and sat on the toilet seat because my bladder felt full, but once again I fell to my knees and let the tide of vomit roll over my tongue. That went on for what seemed like an hour or more. When I was able to leave the bathroom, Kingston was there to lead me back to my room.

The room was spinning. I tried to go to sleep, but my ears started ringing. The ringing wasn't strident, but it was annoying. Whatever was happening to my body, it was apparently out of my control, but I was fighting with everything I had not to vomit or pee in the bed. I rolled from one side to the other, I sat on the edge of the bed, I sat on the floor, and I stood in the corner in the darkness. I laid down again.

Kingston knew he wasn't allowed in the room, but he crossed the threshold, licked my hand and went back out to his post.

The next morning, I was feeling a little better when Staci came into the room to tell me to get dressed for my radiation treatment. She asked me how I was feeling, and I lied and said okay. I was not going to say anything to her about the vomiting. At that point I was going to keep it as secret as a teenager with bulimia.

As I was taking my shower, I looked down and saw the feeding tube dangling from my stomach. I hadn't focused on it since it was 'installed' and I started to wonder when I would need it.

The shower was cleansing and soothing as I washed away the vomit on my chest and feet that remained from the night before. I brushed my teeth and my little bit of hair. I was half-dressed when a wave of nausea hit me. I stepped on Kingston as I ran to the bathroom. He yelped but followed me to the door. Staci was still upstairs getting dressed and didn't hear anything. Nothing was in my stomach, but the retching required a sacrifice, so my stomach gave up its bile. It was sour, bitter, and burned as it spewed from my mouth and brought tears to my eyes. The good thing was that it passed quickly. By the time Staci came down the stairs, I recovered and was ready to go. As we headed for the door, I looked at Kingston, and he seemed relieved that he was off duty and could get rest.

***

After the radiation treatment, we stopped by to see Charles. He was doing so much better after five weeks of treatment and was glad to see us. I told him Staci was leaving soon and that Debbie was coming. Staci showed him the caregiver schedule, and he was glad to see that his sisters jumped in to help.

"I am counting down the days until I can come home for a while. My doctor allows me to leave the building for thirty minutes a day to sit in the sun and get some fresh air if I wear a mask. I am dreaming of pizza and a home-cooked meal."

***

As we were driving home, Staci asked if I wanted to stop for food. I said no, and that I would eat some soup when I got home. By the time we got there, I was exhausted. She went to visit a friend who lived nearby.

I got a blanket, wrapped it around me, and started what would become a daily routine for many months. I called it "cocooning." Once I was inside the blanket, I would turn on the TV and watch "Big Cat Diary." I wouldn't talk or interact. Sometimes I would doze off, but mostly, I would stare off into space. When the show was over, I would go into my room.

I heated up the soup and hoped I could get it down with a few crackers and some tea. I thought maybe if I didn't eat a heavy meal my nausea wouldn't be so severe. I went into the room to lay down, and within minutes I ran to the bathroom. I could see the undigested crackers and noodles floating in the bowl. I flushed them away along with any hope of eating food anytime soon.

I hid my secret for a few more days until the smell of food cooking, soaps, perfumes, deodorants, shampoo, hair spray, toothpaste, coffee and all the aromas of a normal life made me sick. I started carrying my little green bags everywhere I went. It became more important for me to bring those than my purse. I didn't need money, a driver's license, keys, or makeup. I needed to vomit, and it could happen at any time and place. Once again, I was ashamed and embarrassed about my lack of control.

Projectile vomiting is like having a bowel movement in public. It is loud, smelly, toxic, and feral.

Staci relinquished her post and Debbie came in like a whirling dervish. She was, in her words, "On a divine mission." She informed her Bishop that she was going to Atlanta to help us and asked that the church stand in corporate prayer for us. Debbie was a prayer warrior and declared to all that we would defeat this cancer. When she arrived, she had a large suitcase that looked like it could hold enough clothes for a month-long stay, but I knew Staci said each person was on duty for a week so that they would not burn out. When she saw me sitting on the couch looking thin and frail, she began to cry and pray.

"Don't worry, God's grace and mercy would see you through," she said through her tears.

Stevie had just lugged her suitcase upstairs when she asked him to bring it back down.

She pulled it into my room, and it was full of books, sermon cassettes, religious DVDs, vocal and instrumental praise music, and a bottle of anointing oil.

Debbie took the oil that had been prayed over by her Bishop and put it on my forehead, on the tumor, my shoulders, my hands and my feet, while praying and singing. Sometimes she was speaking softly; other times she was yelling loudly at the devil and cancer to leave my body. In some way, it was an exorcism, and in many ways, it was my dearest friend pouring out all the love and faith that she had. When she was exhausted, she retired to her room, and Kingston took up his post.

* * *

The next morning, I had my radiation appointment and a blood test. My nausea was starting to subside, and the frequency of the urge to vomit had lessened.

Debbie had a degree in Medical Technology. This proved helpful when it came time to interpret the results of my blood test. When

83

the nurse was going over the numbers, I couldn't understand the impact or importance of what she was saying, but Debbie was able to translate it for me. She told me the chemotherapy and my inability to eat had lowered my blood count. It was expected, but my ability to fight off any opportunistic infection was diminished.

When we got to the radiation treatment, Greg let her walk to the back to see the machine and mask. She said a quick prayer and returned to the waiting room.

As we were leaving, she stopped and pointed to the name of the center above the door.

"What does that say?" she asked.

"Winship Cancer Center," I whispered.

"Girlfriend, don't you see it, you are on the "Winning Ship," she exclaimed.

"You and Charles are going to make it through this storm."

I smiled. I wanted to laugh, but my throat hurt.

Before we left, she asked if I wanted to see Charles. I was exhausted and said no. She was driving Brooke's car with the GPS, and she let it guide us back with one stop at the grocery store. Debbie wanted to cook dinner for the family and to clean up Brooke's house. I was glad to get home. I felt a need to cocoon and did not want to be outside.

* * *

There were two big boxes in front of the house, and she asked me if I was expecting them. I said no.

I got my blanket and started my ritual. Kingston acknowledged Debbie with his jumping and nuzzling on her and promptly took his position at my feet. Debbie made me some broth, Jell-O, and tea. It was becoming increasingly difficult to swallow. I had been to see a swallowing specialist when I was evaluated, and she told me to expect this and gave me exercises to practice because the radiation treatments would weaken my swallowing muscles. Once again, I couldn't imagine what she was talking about and, with everything else that was happening, I gave those exercises no thought.

Bria came home and was glad to have a homemade meal. She was in her last few days of the school year and was looking forward to summer. She was concerned Kingston was spending too much time with me. Brooke explained to her that studies indicated dogs can smell cancer and she thought that maybe Kingston could smell mine and felt sorry for me.

"Mema, I'm sorry, I was getting a little jealous because since you've been here, he doesn't come to my room anymore or lay at my feet."

I thanked her for understanding and sharing Kingston with me.

Stevie and Brooke were happy for the meal that Debbie prepared. When Stevie brought the boxes in Brooke opened them, it was a two-month supply of my liquid nutrition and instructions to begin the feeding tube. Debbie said based on my blood test, it arrived right on time. I was to have three to six cans a day along with equal amounts of water.

I went into my room and closed the door. I needed a minute to accept this next step. I knew this was coming and now it was here in two big boxes. I looked at the feeding tube and thought again how alien it was. I also thought babies come into the world with the ability to suckle and swallow and as of that moment, I could do neither.

Brooke and Debbie knocked on the door. Brooke was carrying the bag of syringes and pads and a box of gloves. Debbie had three cans of the nutrition and a pitcher of water. I laid back and closed my eyes and listened to Brooke instruct Debbie. Suddenly, I felt the warm flow of the liquid in my stomach. It started filling up all the empty spaces that I had been ignoring. Debbie said a prayer and pushed down on the syringe and slowly released it. She followed it with water which felt cold and tickled. My body was immediately grateful and responded with a surge of belching and gas.

Brooke asked how I felt, and I told her much better. She said goodnight and left to be with her family. Debbie stayed and flushed the feeding tube and changed the bandage around the hole in my stomach. She rubbed more oil on me, read me scriptures, and held my hand as I went to sleep with a full belly.

* * *

Charles called early in the morning and asked if he could hitch a ride with us after my radiation appointment. After six weeks, he was discharged and excited to come home for ten days before returning for further treatment.

When I finished, we went over to Charles' room. He was packed and ready to go. It was good to see him in regular clothes, though they were hanging off him due to his considerable weight loss. This was the first time Debbie had seen him, and before we left the room, she prayed over him and thanked God for his improvement and continued healing. She promised to anoint him with the oil when we got home.

When we got home, Charles called and had pizzas delivered, much to the delight of Bria. He asked me if I wanted pepperoni or cheese. It was at that moment I realized how out of touch we were. Charles didn't know that I couldn't swallow and that I was now dependent on the feeding tube. Debbie showed him the cans and told him about the syringe and the whole process. He looked at her like she arrived from another planet.

I was ready to cocoon, but before I could do that, I grabbed his hand and we went into the bedroom. I lifted my shirt and showed him the tube and the feeding supply set up next to the bed. He bent down and kissed my stomach near the tube.

Brooke and Stevie were glad to see Charles and celebrated the progress he made. Debbie came down to join the celebration. It was time to give me a feeding and to show Charles the procedure.

He watched closely and said, "I know there are going to be other caregivers coming, but when I am able, I want to take care of my wife."

Debbie prayed over us and put oil on Charles' head. She reminded me that she only had two more days of duty and then she was going to spend a few days with her son, Marcus, who lived in Atlanta.

Charles' and I snuggled for the first time in months. He was cautious not to touch my feeding tube, and we were hyper-aware of germs and cleanliness. I was glad that my nausea abated and that he missed those horrific episodes. We were together now, and there was a moment of peace. We went to sleep holding on to that peace and to each other.

Debbie was leaving and said she was on the schedule to return in five weeks. She promised to call and check if I needed her to come back sooner. I missed her as soon as she walked out of the door. We had been friends for more than forty years, but now I saw her like the angel she always was as she fluttered off with her big red suitcase.

***

Charles and I spent the weekend catching up with each other's doctor's visits, treatments, and blood tests. To someone from the outside, it would sound like a strange conversation, but for us it was necessary. Charles didn't have a clue of what I was going through. He had not seen the machine or mask associated with the radiation, nor had he been to the infusion center for chemotherapy. His chemo treatments did not cause him the extreme nausea that I was experiencing. The only thing we had in common was the tingling in our hands and feet. He had a hearty appetite, but I could not eat. He noticed the discoloration in my neck from the radiation and said that it looked like the tumor was smaller. He would see everything soon—I was going to have my second round of chemo and my tenth radiation treatment.

***

Charles was home and able to help care for me. Staci asked my friend Lois if she could provide transportation for us. Lois lived more than thirty miles south, and Winship was thirty miles north of the house. She was driving more than one hundred and twenty-miles round trip to help me. I was beyond grateful. I knew her elderly father had prostate cancer and that she and her sister Monica were taking turns giving him care, and yet she found time for me.

When we got to the center, she and Charles were shocked at the condition of the people in the radiation waiting room but were more upset when they walked back with me and saw the machine and mask. After radiation, we headed to chemo. After a short wait, the tech called my name, and we walked to the bay. The nurse said I would be there for two hours and that they could go to lunch. Charles was reluctant, but I insisted that they go.

As I waited for my nurse, I noticed the number of men caregivers. Whether they were husbands with their wives, a father with a daughter, a son with his mother or father or whatever the relationship, in the center they took on what traditionally is considered a female role. They were arranging blankets, wiping faces, holding bottles up to eager mouths, feeding snacks, and stroking the hands or cheeks of their loved one.

Lorna, the nurse, started my IV. She was delightful and upbeat. "I'm going to give you this chemo, but you remember that true healing comes from love. While you are going through this only surround yourself with people that love you. No negativity, no stress or anger." Lorna whispered as she helped me to get comfortable.

I dozed off while the chemo trickled, but I woke to a cacophony of moans, heaves, and hurls again. I remembered how sick I was for five days after my last chemo and prayed that I wouldn't be as sick this time. My doctor prescribed a patch for me to wear that would lessen the nausea. I felt hopeful that this time would be different.

As soon as I was finished, Lois said we needed to leave so that she didn't have to sit in rush hour traffic. I started to cocoon in the car on the way home.

***

By the time we got to the house, I couldn't tell Lois goodbye. I barely got through the door when nausea walloped me. I rushed to the bathroom and let it go, all the liquid sustenance Charles gave me that morning was now flowing like Niagara Falls.

Charles and Kingston stood outside the door, both whimpering in sympathy with me and each other. Because of his weakened immune system and the toxicity of my vomit, Charles couldn't come near until I disinfected the area.

He kept asking if I was okay, but I was hurling and gagging too much to answer. When it subsided, I was soaking wet with sweat and too dizzy to walk. Stevie came home as I was trying to move, and he helped me to bed. Charles put on a mask, wiped me down with a warm cloth and changed my clothes. He got the feeding kit out and, despite my protest, managed to get water and sustenance in the tube.

I had a patch around my tube, a bandage where I had the IV, a patch for nausea and a patch for pain. I felt like a used tire with patches everywhere but still leaking air and going flat.

***

90

The next day we made it to our appointments. Lois seemed overwhelmed with two patients. While his blood transfusion revitalized Charles, I could barely stand. I was still nauseous and had used multiple green bags that morning and at one point, I needed Lois to pull over so that I wouldn't let go in the car.

* * *

Once home, Charles jumped into action taking care to feed me and rub aloe vera on my neck which was now showing signs of severe burns. Bria went to visit family in South Carolina for a few weeks. Brooke and Stevie met for dinner after work and came home later than usual. I was in the shower when I heard them talking to Charles. I felt weak, but I wanted the water to cleanse and soothe me. I put on my pajamas and headed towards the bedroom. I was dizzy and couldn't feel my legs. I blacked out as Brooke walked into the room. She caught me and I remained conscious just long enough to hear her scream.

"Call 911! Mommy is down!"

When I regained consciousness, the EMT had started an IV and was asking me my name. I could hear him, but I couldn't respond. I heard Brooke saying stage four cancer, I saw Stevie pacing outside the door, and I saw Charles standing over me with new tears in his eyes.

They wanted to carry me to the nearest emergency room, but Brooke insisted that they take me to Emory Hospital. It was after midnight when they admitted me to the hospital. An exhausted Brooke and Stevie drove back home; they had to go to work in a few hours.

Charles stayed in the hospital and slept in the recliner in my room. When the staff changed shifts, the nurse was shocked to see Charles.

"Mr. Ross, what are you doing here? I thought we sent you home."

When he explained the situation, she shook her head and backed out of the room.

My doctor said I was severely dehydrated, and my blood pressure and counts were frightfully low. I was taken over to Winship for my radiation treatment and given more glucose and hydration. Charles had his infusion there at the same time. I was taken back to the hospital and discharged with instructions to increase feedings and water. I was prescribed another series of patches to be worn two at a time for nausea and another for pain.

I was suffering.

My tongue was black.

My throat burned, no matter how much pain medication I was given.

Nausea would begin at any time, and my spirit was waning.

Charles was going back to the hospital in a few days to resume his treatment for two weeks. He needed care instead of serving as my caregiver. It was taking a toll on him.

* * *

Charles' sister, Shirley, arrived from Virginia to take her post. She was full of energy and ready to work. She said she was praying and crying on the plane ride and wanted to help Brooke as much as possible while she was there. Once she got settled and talked to Brooke and Charles, she came into the bedroom.

She told me to pray.

"Prayer is the lifeline between the one who needs help and the hearer."

She was eager to learn how to use the feeding tube, and Charles instructed her as she fed me. She also wanted to see Winship and told Brooke she wanted to help around the house. Brooke gave her the nickname, "Busy," and we all agreed it fit her perfectly.

Stevie had a few days off, so he became our driver. Charles was re-admitted to the hospital. I had my radiation appointments and a scheduled Cat Scan of the tumor. Shirley went with Charles. Stevie stayed with me.

Shirley was sad that Charles wouldn't be coming home with us. When we got home, she fed me and prepared dinner. I was falling asleep before she finished but I could sense her silent tears as I went out. When her time was up, I knew I was going to miss "Busy." Shirley was another angel who could have flown in on her own wings but took a plane instead. She took such good care of us, and she had a fondness for Kingston. With Charles and Shirley gone, I felt alone, until I heard Kingston back on his post outside my door.

Early the next morning as I stepped out of the shower, I noticed a patch of hair on the bathroom floor. I looked in the mirror and saw the bald spot. When Stevie came down, I asked him to shave my head completely bald. He looked away, held his breath, and did it.

93

I was getting weaker, and I could no longer look in the mirror. I didn't recognize that human that looked back. It was frail, bald, with cracking skin, dark eyes, and sunken cheeks, no smile, no gender, no Bari.

I was only halfway through my treatments, and I was scared to think about what the other half would bring.

Lois' sister, Monica, became my driver for another week of radiation. Monica was low key and calm. I loved her for it. She wanted to know that I was going to fight and not give up. She lost her husband to cancer eight months before and was still grieving. Yet, she was making time to help me. She also was driving more than hundred miles round trip to get me to my appointments. I was so humbled and grateful for another angel and thanked God daily for the blessings of love.

* * *

The fireworks were brilliant in the hot July 4th night sky. Brooke wrapped a blanket around me. We sat on her lawn watching the sky turn white, then blue and bright red. She drew the blanket closer around my shoulders.

"How are you feeling, Mommy?"

I looked up at the spinner as it rose in the air and burst into a comet that streaked across the sky before I responded.

"Weak and nauseous."

She looked up as the whirling fireworks exploded into a waterfall.

"Stephen and I are pregnant," she told me.

94

I shivered and vomited.

They had been trying to have a baby for a year. On the outside, I was so happy for them and excited. I could see that over the next few months, as cancer and the treatment did battle in my body, that she would blossom as the baby grew in her body. In a few weeks, the differences were clear. I was losing weight rapidly; Brooke was getting bigger.

My skin was being burned and charred. Her skin was glowing. I was bald. Her hair was growing thicker and stronger. I was losing my memory. She was multi-tasking work, taking care of her family, me, and Charles. I was losing my ability to talk.

My tongue was black, and my throat was fiery red. She was laughing and sharing her news with everyone. I was losing contact with my husband. Her husband would put his hands on her growing bump at every opportunity.

As the fireworks ended with a sonic boom, Brooke helped me into the room and gave me a feeding and put me to bed as if she was practicing for the new baby.

* * *

Brooke's birthday was coming up and Stevie planned a much-needed getaway. Staci came in a few days before they were to leave so that she could take Brooke on a "sister date." I am sure Brooke told Staci about my deterioration but seeing it had to have been shocking for her. The rapid twenty-pound weight loss in less than a month, the bald head, the radiation burns, the slow movements, the mental confusion, and the emotional withdrawal was not something she had ever imagined her mother going through. Her face said it all when she came into the room.

Staci looked at me in disbelief and sat on the edge of the bed.

The only time I wasn't in bed was when I was going to Winship. I was no longer "cocooning," watching TV, or even attempting to read or write. My doctor said I had "Chemo Brain," which was another side effect of the treatment, the pain medicine, and the stress. Once again, I was ashamed that I couldn't remember what happened the previous day, that I was stumbling for words or that I couldn't read and comprehend a simple paragraph, so I withdrew to my bedroom where I felt safe.

I found a peculiar kind of loneliness when I was suffering. It was peaceful and painful at the same time. The peace was that I appreciated not having to explain anything to anyone. The pain was that I wanted to be understood or affirmed by others who had no idea of what I was experiencing.

Brooke and Stevie left for their trip, and Staci took over the caregiving. I had doctors, scans, and radiation appointments.

Staci brought a gift bag into the room and said it was from her friend, Katrice. I've known Katrice since she and Staci were on the girl's high school track team. When I opened the bag, I saw twenty different scarves of all colors, lengths, shapes, and sizes. I was touched that she thought of me and took the time to shop for me. Another angel with a small gift that meant so much.

* * *

"Staci, I'm not sure I want to continue these treatments. The chemo has me vomiting, the radiation has me burning and in pain," I cried.

She looked at me earnestly and said, "Mommy, it's not the treatment. It's the CANCER."

"No, I wasn't sick, weak, fatigued, bald, burned, and ugly until I started these treatments."

Staci didn't argue. She applied the aloe vera to my neck, fed me, cleaned my face, and closed the door. She didn't like dogs, and Kingston knew that. He instinctively waited until she went upstairs to take his place at the door, whimpering loudly.

When I quieted down, I realized that she was right. It was the CANCER. It invaded me and laid claim to my body. It was putting up a steadfast and deliberate fight against the regiment of medicines and procedures being sent to battle it.

It was declaring, "I got here first. I was gaining ground at my own pace, and I have no intention of going anywhere. No chemo or radiation or anything else is going to stop me. You read the statistics. I win more than I lose at Stage 4B."

I recognized that Cancer is an enemy that wants destruction and nothing less. The body is the first strike in the war. Fighting cancer is not a battle; it is a war that is all consuming. It demands all your resources be they physical, material, financial, emotional, or spiritual.

97

The next day, when Staci and I arrived at my appointment, the Radiologist-Oncologist had good news for us. After three weeks of treatment, the tumor was shrinking or, at least, wasn't growing. He recognized that I was in constant pain and when he looked at my tongue, and down my throat, he said, while it looked horrible, it meant that the treatment was working. He increased my pain medicine with another patch.

The news buoyed Staci. After we left his office, she called Brooke. I heard what he said, but it didn't affect me the same way. All I could think of was that I had four more weeks of treatment and I was already at what I thought was my physical limit.

We went to see "The Captain," who confirmed that the radiation and chemo were working but reminded us that additional surgery might be necessary to ensure that all the cancer is eliminated.

Staci was writing and asking questions. I refused to participate in the conversation. I was trying to get through the chemo and radiation. I couldn't think about a future surgery,

As we were leaving, Staci asked if I wanted to see Charles. I said no. On the drive home, Staci asked why I wasn't happy about the fact that the tumor was responding to the treatment and why I was surly with the ENT. I decided I wasn't going to talk to her either.

I was in so much pain that it hurt to swallow my saliva. I had patches everywhere and yet no relief. I had beautiful, loving caregivers. What I lacked was comfort. People who looked at me looked away because they could see the horrible physical effects of Stage 4B cancer and its treatment.

The next day, we went to see the Medical Oncologist who had more good news; I may not need the next round of chemotherapy, my blood tests had reached the lowest point, and since the tumor was shrinking, a third round may not be necessary. Staci was writing. I was looking at the wall. The nurse said the doctor prescribed a new patch for nausea, that it was a clinical trial, and if I agreed to use it, the company would send it directly to the house. I nodded yes, but I didn't believe it would work.

* * *

We went over to the hospital to pick up Charles. He was looking forward to being discharged, but when we got there, he was sitting in the chair in pajamas looking dejected. They discovered that he had an infection and a low-grade fever, so they were going to keep him and give him antibiotics for two more days. Staci tried to cheer him up by telling him the good news from my doctors. It worked. Charles smiled and hugged me. He complimented me on the beautiful headscarf I was wearing. Staci told him Katrice sent me a gift box of scarves.

Charles asked me why I wasn't talking to him, I said nothing. I felt as though my words were useless. No one could understand what I was feeling and since it hurt so much to talk, I wouldn't bother.

Staci was getting burnt out from caregiving. On the last day before Brooke and Stevie were to return, she told me she was going to meet one of her college friends for dinner. After she left and I was alone, I thought maybe if I wrote I would feel better. I tried to go up the steps to the second floor to get paper and realized that I didn't have the strength to make it all the way to the top. After the fifth step, I turned around and decided to go back to my bedroom. I made it to the couch before I collapsed. Kingston came and sat on my feet and licked my hand. I laid there with my little green bag until Staci came home and put me to bed.

The next morning Staci said,

"Mommy, before I leave, I have a question, and I don't know if you know the answer, but where are Mr. Charles' son and daughter?"

I shrugged my shoulders because I didn't know the answer. She didn't think it was fair that all of this was on her and Brooke, and that they didn't call to offer any assistance or even to say thank you for being there for their father. Brooke and Stevie were disappointed about the lack of support from Charles' children.

With all that was happening, it wasn't something I thought about, but I couldn't deny that she had a point. When Charles came home, I was going to ask him because Staci was right. It didn't seem fair, but for me, nothing seemed "fair" anymore. I was already in agonizing pain, and this was another kind of pain piling on.

Charles' infection was stubborn and the projected two days turned into six before he was discharged. The next week was hectic because there was not one consistent driver. Charles was going to be my caregiver and Brooke was putting together a crew of drivers from members of her church.

She said these were people she had confidence in, and I should trust them.

"Mommy, please be pleasant and not grouchy. They want to help."

Since I was barely able to speak and or move, I didn't have a choice but to obey.

I recognized the first driver as the young lady who told me how blessed I was to be chosen to have cancer. She said her sister was a recent survivor of breast cancer, she realized that Brooke needed a village to help her, and that she was here to do her part. I wanted to ask her about her comment, but I was still not talking and the "chemo brain" was in full effect. I whispered thank you as we headed to my twentieth radiation treatment. I could barely walk, so she pushed me in a wheelchair to the waiting arms of my favorite tech. He tried to make me laugh. I had no laughs in me; my entire existence was pain.

* * *

When she drove me home, Charles helped me out of the car and carried me to bed. He had the feeding tools set up and was ready before my head touched the pillow. He was efficient and moved carefully to make sure he didn't miss a step. I was washing up daily because of all the patches, the feeding tube and feared the water hitting my skin, but today I wanted a shower. He went into the bathroom and made sure that the water temperature and force were mild. He gently removed each patch and led me to the bathroom.

I thought he was going to grab my arm to make sure I didn't slip or faint. Instead, he stepped into the shower with me and held me with one hand and bathed me gently with the other. He stood between me and the direct hit of the water and used the cloth to create a soft drizzle. My right side was charred from beneath my cheek to the top of my breast, and all the skin in that area hurt. Each of us had

101

varying degrees of neuropathy in our feet and hands; yet, he was the caregiver because I had no care to give. He applied the aloe vera, gave me more water through the tube, reapplied the patches, and put me to bed.

Three days later, Britta was replaced by another member of the church. Her name was Millie. She was a nurse at Emory Hospital and came to pick me up on her day off.

I was grateful that despite Millie's busy life, she was giving her time. She knew several of the nurses and they treated her with great respect. When she took me home, she told Charles to rest, and she took over the feeding and changed my patches and bandages. She read the reports and said she knew I was in pain, but that the treatments were having the intended effect. She encouraged me to be patient, keep fighting and keep praying.

Millie came many times to check on me, and she also made it a point to visit Charles when he was in the hospital and she was at work. She was another angel who floated into our lives on the wings of love.

The practical things still must be done, and these were left to Charles when he was home, our friend Beverly in Phoenix called saying that the HOA wanted my car and his truck moved immediately and that we needed to get our stuff out of the condo since it was apparent we wouldn't be coming back. Bev said she was willing to pack our stuff up and take it to storage.

Charles told her to choose anything she wanted and to call our grandson David who was in his second year at Arizona State University to give him my car and any furniture he wanted. I asked her to keep my books and anything I might deem irreplaceable. She did as we asked and instead of putting things in storage because she knew we didn't have the monthly fee, she kept over fifty boxes of our stuff in the living room of her condo. No doubt she was sent from heaven. There were also so many cards and letters piled up in our bedroom that I didn't have the desire or the strength to read. Charles opened each one and read the verses and prayers that each one offered. Many of the names I didn't recognize because they were members of Brooke's church.

His niece, Bearly, sent us several beautiful cards and his cousin Pat who sent cards for each occasion had outdone herself in the beauty and heartfelt cards that she sent.

Charles called Dad to let him know how we were doing. He contacted Reverend Perry and thanked him for his comfort. In the mail were two gas cards, one for each of us, for a hundred dollars from the American Cancer Society.

Staci called to say Traci was next on the schedule, but she wouldn't be able to stay a week.

Traci was on the plane to Atlanta when my doctor put me in the hospital for pain management. When she arrived, I was on so much medication that I didn't know she was there. Charles said she stood by the bed and cried

"Oh, my poor sister, look at her."

She had several questions, but he couldn't answer them. She was there to help, and there was nothing to do. Charles suggested that she get a warm cloth and wipe my face and she did so with tears falling from her eyes.

Charles decided to spend the night in the chair. He gave her directions to Brooke's house. She was disappointed and distraught. She had no idea how bad things were. Her hopes of going back to Cincinnati with good news for Dad were dashed against the morphine drip that was hanging from my pole.

ANGELS
TO THE RESCUE

My pain had become excruciating to the point that I couldn't function. My team of doctors decided to admit me to the hospital to get it under control. I never heard of a pain specialist, but when he came to the room to explain what his role was, I was hopeful that he had some relief with my name on it. He immediately ordered a morphine pump that allowed me to push a button and have morphine delivered in measured doses up to three times an hour. We tried it for two days, while it made me sleep it did not reduce my pain. I was feeding through the tube, but instead of having it through a syringe, I was tethered to a machine that continuously pumped the liquid.

Despite being in the hospital, I still received my daily radiation treatment. By the third day, he decided that I needed the most potent painkiller they could offer. It was typically used to keep terminal patients "comfortable" until they made their transition. It was carefully monitored and could only be given for a few days. It gave me some relief, but it was clear that I couldn't continue to use it for fear of addiction.

Charles told me that Traci came to visit every day while she was in town. I regret that I couldn't remember her being there, but I've known she was an angel since the day she was born.

I was discharged from the hospital after five days. When Stevie came to pick me up, he couldn't look at me. Though he was gentle with every move he made to help me into the wheelchair and into the car, he couldn't make eye contact. I knew he didn't want to cry.

I imagined I reminded him of his beloved mother in the final stages of her cancer fight, and it was too much for a powerful Ninja to bear. Later, Brooke told me he cried many nights when they were alone and recalled the memories of his mother's battle.

When I got home, there was an electric feeding machine in my room like the one at the hospital. The nutritionist ordered it and said that because I was losing weight and my blood tests were coming back at the lowest levels, I needed to be on the machine to maintain a consistent level of sustenance to help me through the last ten radiation treatments.

Charles was doing well and was looking forward to Regina's return. He was buoyed even more. She was bringing his sisters Polly and Odell for a week-long visit.

When they arrived at the house, I was in bed. I could hear their voices as they were complimenting Charles on how well he looked and how blessed he was to be getting the best treatment.

As I lay there with the machine whirring and clicking, I didn't want them to come into the room. I felt so ugly and ashamed. I lost more than thirty pounds, and my skin looked reptilian. My eyes were sunken into my skull like two bottomless pits, and my gums receded from my teeth, so my smile was garish. I frightened myself to the point that I would brush my teeth in the dark.

Charles asked if I wanted to come out to the living room or if they could come in and see me. I opted to get up and join them and let them see everything. He helped me get dressed, and when I hobbled out of the door and turned the corner, I saw the look in their eyes. They were not prepared for what they saw.

Regenia said that she and Polly would be staying at a nearby hotel and would drive Charles and me to our appointments and would help with hands-on care. Odell said she would be staying with her daughter in a suburb of Atlanta, but she would catch up with us from time to time. Odell said something that I love and respect her for, "Bari, I can't do hands-on. I am too squeamish and nervous."

I wish more people would have been forthcoming and honest instead of turning away or ignoring us. Kingston was sitting on my feet, as they were ready to leave. They wanted to hug me, but he wouldn't budge, so Regenia told him, "That's okay, big boy. You stay on your side. I'll stay on mine."

Charles' sisters heights barely averaged five feet. But everyone who came with me for my radiation treatments was five feet six or taller. My tech was always trying to make me smile so when I introduced him to my sisters-in-law he said, "Mrs. Ross they're sitting on the couch, but their feet aren't touching the floor."

I looked back over my shoulder and smiled. He was right. From that day to now, though they are all older than me, I call them my "little" sisters.

Polly had years of experience in caregiving as a home healthcare aid, and she was so gentle and loving when helping me. There were times when I was surly or snappy, and she would try to soothe me and get through the task. There was one day when Charles and Regenia ran errands and left her with me. The phone rang, and it was Debbie. Polly told her I couldn't talk because my throat was hurting, and I was only saying a few words when necessary.

Debbie replied,

"Just put the phone up to her ear. I'll do all the talking!"

Polly did what Debbie asked. When Regenia and Charles came home, Polly laughed,

"I've never heard anything like that in all my years. Most people say, I'll call back when they are feeling better, but not Debbie."

* * *

After a few days of appointments, Regenia decided it was time to do something different. Odell rejoined us. Charles received great news on his improving blood counts. It was a cause for celebration at the restaurant of his choice. I was feeling weak and nauseous, but I didn't want to spoil the fun.

When we left the hospital, Regenia headed to the famous Perimeter Mall of Atlanta. It was a hot day in mid-July. Because of the radiation

108

treatments, I couldn't be out in the sun without a big hat and plenty of sunscreen. Regenia left us in the car and ran into the store and bought both. She treated Charles to a mini shopping spree. He was happy to be showered with the love and attention they were giving him, and I was delighted to see him smiling.

After shopping, we headed to a restaurant called Mimi's. I couldn't eat or drink, but I thought maybe I could sit and watch them enjoy.

After they placed their orders, I started to feel light-headed. I laid my head against Charles' shoulder and took a few breaths, but when the waitress brought the food to the table, the smells hit me hard.

Despite my neuropathy and weakness, I bolted to the ladies' room. I had my green bag with me which caught most of it, but I still fell to my knees and hugged the bowl.

When the wave passed, I went and laid down on the backseat of the car with the air conditioning on while they hurriedly finished lunch. Regenia opened the door,

"Look what I have for you. You didn't think I was going to treat everyone to lunch and forget about you."

When I saw what she had, I cried. It was two cans of sustenance, two bottles of water, the syringe, towels, gloves, pads, and patches. She drove to a far corner of the parking lot and found a shade tree where she parked and let the others out of the car. She laid me down, fed me, patched me up, and drove home.

We were sorry to see our three angels fly away. The merry-go-round of caregivers was on its second and third rotation for some of its riders.

Charles returned to the hospital for his treatment for two weeks, and Staci returned. The doctors agreed that I couldn't tolerate any more chemo. I needed to finish the last week of radiation.

I was in pain and my "chemo brain" was in high gear. My short-term memory was non-existent and my ability to comprehend time and space collapsed into a dark void. I didn't know the time of day or the day of the week. I woke up one morning and saw black ashes all around my pillow. I thought someone who smoked must have come into the room and dropped ashes in my bed, but no one in the house smoked.

In a moment of clarity, I realized it was the skin off my neck, chest, and shoulder. I picked it up, and it blew away. As painful as it was, I touched my neck, and the burned skin was coming off in sheets like thin tissue paper. I lay there praying for a slight wind to come and blow the rest of me away. At the end of the week, my Radiologist-Oncologist announced that I successfully completed my treatments and that I would see him weekly for the next six weeks as he monitored my recovery. I would also need to have another series of scans. He seemed pleased and said that the tumor responded favorably to the treatments. He recommended plenty of rest and water. He hugged me and offered my mask, "Some people like to keep them as souvenirs."

I could barely speak, but I was able to tell him to throw mine away; this was not a trip from which I wanted any souvenirs.

Staci was happy to inform family and friends that my treatments were complete. She sent an email and made a few calls before we left. Brooke said she didn't know much about the recovery period, but if I

110

continued to follow the program, I should be better by the fall.

It was July 31, and the fall seemed as distant as June 8th, the day I started my treatments seven weeks earlier. Both were far away from where I was now.

Over the next few days, congratulatory cards, letters, and phone calls poured in, and Staci was responding to each one. Three of Staci's college friends, thinking the end of treatment meant I could eat, sent a beautiful Edible Arrangement of fruit. I couldn't swallow, but I enjoyed the beauty. I fed some of it to Kingston so that he could celebrate and was surprised he liked pineapple.

The only voice I wanted to hear was my father's. He frequently called to check on me and always told Brooke to let me know but not to disturb me. The idea of hearing me moan in pain was more than either of us could stand. Regardless of my pain, on this day I wanted to hear his voice. Staci called him for me. I started crying before I put the phone to my ear. He was calm and measured and said he and Mary prayed for Charles and me every day. He told me to fight to get well so that I could visit him.

Charles came home to the job of full-time caregiver. Since I didn't have to go to the center daily, we didn't need transportation, and the machine was pumping in the nutrition. Charles was free to handle other things. His energy level was low. Some days, we both slept holding hands. Millie would call and come by to check on us. Many times, she would send Charles out to walk Kingston and get some fresh air while she sat with me. She told him how important it was for him to get exercise so that he could get stronger. He had to wear

111

his mask, and it was a double blessing because it kept the high levels of allergens out of his system as well as any germs. His number one objective was not to get any infections that would set back his recovery.

His immune system was weak, and any infection could become lethal. Charles assumed the role of germ-fighter. He washed and changed our sheets daily, he scrubbed and disinfected our bathroom twice a day, he wiped down my feeding machine daily, he wore gloves and his mask to handle my green bags and immediately took them outside to the garbage can far away from the house. He only ate on paper plates and used plastic utensils. If we were in a car and someone sneezed, he would have the window down to let out the germs before they could hang in the air. With his hair loss from chemo, I thought, "He is the true Mr. Clean."

***

It was early August, and Debbie called to say she was coming to do another round of caregiving and to celebrate my birthday. The next morning, we all loaded into Brooke's car, making our way to the hospital. Charles and I were in the back seat wearing masks. Brooke was driving when suddenly, blue-flashing lights appeared in the mirror, and a police cruiser was behind us. Brooke pulled over to let him pass, the policeman pulled up next to us blocking the intersection and signaled Brooke to stop. The officer sauntered over to our car, peered into the rear where we were seated, and barked, "So where are you folks going?"

When Brooke explained she was driving us to Emory Hospital, the police ordered Brooke to step out of the car. Brooke complied. Surely, he could see two obviously ill people in the car, unless he presumed, we were robbers with hospital masks on.

The officer came back to the car and said,

"Your registration tag has expired and I'm going to have to cite you."

Debbie interjected, "Sir, we're trying to get my sister and brother-in-law to the hospital for cancer treatment. Do you understand this was an honest oversight? Can't you help us due to the circumstances?"

He looked at us again and mellowed.

"Well, if you get this taken care of today, I'll let you go. If you don't, your vehicle will be impounded."

"Yes sir, I will."

We dropped Brooke off at work and went to our appointments. When we finished at Winship, we took Charles home and scurried to get to the DMV before it closed.

I was exhausted. Debbie sat me in a corner and wrapped my blanket around me. She went to the window to conduct the business. She could see I was fading. Brooke wasn't there, and the clerk was not going to let Debbie pay the fee to renew the registration. Debbie was trying to negotiate with her because she gave Brooke her word that she would take care of it and because she didn't want a repeat of what happened that morning with the policeman. I could see them going back and forth in a verbal tug-of-war. I feebly walked over and told Debbie we should let Brooke or Stevie take care of it. Debbie looked at me, and a light bulb went on in her head.

She said to the clerk, "Look, ma'am, I drove my sister here from cancer treatment, and that's when the policeman stopped us. Surely you can have some empathy. I am here from Ohio to help take care of her. Please see if you can assist us."

Once she heard the word cancer and looked at me in my most pitiful state, she stamped the paperwork and issued the new registration.

Sometimes caregiving requires skills other than feeding and tender care; sometimes it needs a strong voice and a determined heart. Debbie has both.

We had a quiet but fun celebration for my birthday. Everyone took a deep sigh of relief that "Operation Keep Mommy and Papa Charles Alive" was working and despite my outward appearance, things were improving. Debbie suggested I try to go to church on Sunday. Brooke said we could sit in the back so that if I needed to leave for any reason, I would be by the door. When I woke up Sunday morning, I was feeling decent. Debbie tied one of the beautiful scarves around my head. I was nervous because I was still having occasional bouts of nausea. I put two of my green bags in my pocket.

We got to the church a little early to ensure that we were in the back row near the door. Brooke talked to the ushers and made sure they knew our concerns.

At one point, I did have to make a quick exit. As soon as I moved one of them gently grabbed my arm and helped me to the bathroom. She patiently waited outside the door. She said her aunt had cancer and carried a green bag with her. So, when she saw me take mine out of my pocket, she knew what to do.

"I'm praying for you, Brooke, and the family. You all have a lot on you right now. God will take care of you," she whispered.

During the service I cried tears of sorrow for the things we had been through and tears of joy for the promise of things to come. As we were leaving The First Lady, Libby, complimented me, "I like the scarf and the earrings, every woman can't wear that and look as refined as you do."

Her compliment made me blush. As much as I like compliments from my husband, hearing these things from another woman was a boost to my diminished self-esteem.

Pastor Pollard walked over and asked how we were doing. Brooke told him that several people in the congregation had been helping us.

Pastor Pollard said a prayer for us and the little new one that was growing inside of Brooke. Many people came to us to extend their good wishes, prayers, offers to cook, to visit, or help in any way. When we left, I thought, here is a church of angels. No wonder Brooke and Stevie feel at home here. They have found the perfect extended family.

* * *

Charles was back on duty. A month passed since my last treatment, and I wasn't close to eating or drinking. The doctor insisted that I increase my water intake. My potassium level was low, which could harm my kidneys. When Charles heard that, I thought he was going to drown me through my tube. He hung bags of water on the feeding machine day and night. I got more exercise from going to the bathroom twenty feet from my bed than from the daily short walks the doctors prescribed.

We were getting stronger, and the doctor reduced my pain medication. Charles' stays in the hospital were getting shorter. However, his outpatient treatment for blood platelets and lumbar punctures remained consistent. A lumbar puncture is like an epidural—instead of blocking pain, it is a direct shot of chemotherapy to the spine to seek out and destroy any leukemia cells that may be forming there.

In mid-September, I went to see the "Captain." Brooke came with me. She was starting to show her baby bump. He congratulated her and told me I had to get well to help Brooke with the newcomer. I hadn't thought about taking care of a baby. It was something I could look forward to doing.

* * *

As in many scenarios in life, there is good news and bad, and it has never made a difference to me which one I hear first, because they each must be dealt with. When the doctor said the tumor was gone, I was reluctant to react. I could see and feel that it was no longer beneath my ear, but since cancer had spread beyond that area, I needed to hear that the cancer was gone.

"To be sure we got all the cancer in the lymph nodes, I need to perform a "radical neck dissection.""

I looked at Brooke's face and saw two big moons.

We had discussed the possibility of surgery in our initial visits, but that seemed like ancient history. I thought that the chemo and radiation defeated the tumor and we were here to declare victory. Instead, he

116

was discussing another major attack using a bombshell weapon that would leave me permanently disfigured.

I was listening, but I could not hear. Brooke was nodding her head to the words that were coming out of his moving lips, which signaled to me that she understood and agreed with him. Chemo brain, fear, and disappointment would not let me accept what he was proposing. As I tried to slip into a safer place, Cancer spoke directly to me.

"I'm not done yet. How many people have had chemo and radiation and didn't beat me? If that were all it took, they would have lived a long life or would still be alive. What makes you think I haven't evolved or adapted to the usual tactics and medicines? I am not giving up. I want you or your husband or you and your husband. I finish what I start. Don't believe even if you have this surgery that this is over."

I slumped down in the chair as I watched the doctor and Brooke talk. My body was beaten down and barely functioning. Every inch of it ached, from my throat to my toes. I had nothing left to negotiate with except my soul, and I sat there questioning its value.

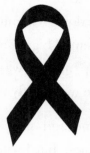

MISSING PARTS

Six weeks later, I was on my way to the operating room with the Captain and his team. Brooke and Charles were in the waiting room.

The night before, Brooke explained to me what the surgery entailed.

"Mommy, the doctor is going to remove lymph nodes, part of a major muscle, and a nerve that will leave you with no feeling on the right side of your body from the top of your ear to the top of your breast. You will have limited range of motion when turning your head and your right shoulder will droop, and your mouth may curve slightly to the right as if you had a stroke. I know it sounds terrible, but we've gone this far, and we've got to be certain that there is no cancer hiding in your lymph nodes."

Charles backed her up, "Honey, listen to Brooke and the doctor. We already know how sneaky Cancer is and we need to make sure it is gone, and if this will help do that, then you must go forth and conquer."

One lone tear fell from my eye, and Charles caught it before it hit my chin.

When the "Captain" came to pre-op, he seemed different. I'd only seen him in a small room doing examinations, interpreting scans, and blood tests. Here he seemed bigger and yet more personal. The operating room was his ship, and he was ready to take it out to the vast open sea of surgery. He was clearly in command.

He put his hand over mine and said, "I know you may not be comfortable with your decision, but I will do my best to take care of you and leave as little damage as possible."

I nodded. I had exhausted the English language of all the words I knew to explain my feelings.

The nurse rolled me towards the operating room. The last thing I saw was Brooke giving me the thumbs up sign and her baby bump pushing against her emerald green top.

The surgery took seven hours, and when I woke up, a nurse was trying to get me off the gurney and on the hospital bed. My head felt like a volcano blast blew the top off. I didn't know if I had a body from my eyes down. And I didn't care. I was trying to separate the fragments of my mind from the lava and put the pieces back together.

I could hear Brooke saying, "Mommy, Mommy" but she was far away. I could hear Charles' voice, but it was being carried away by the lava.

I could hear Cancer laughing, "I told you so, I told you so."

I thought I was in Hell.

I didn't remember anything for two days, and then on the third morning I heard Charles snoring in the chair bed next to me. I recognized the familiar sound of the feeding machine and then the beeping sound of the monitor. I tried to turn my head but couldn't. I tried to speak and nothing came out. I laid in the dark and began purring like a kitten.

The tech came in to take my vital signs, and when she saw my eyes open, she said,

"Well, good morning, Sleeping Beauty."

Charles jumped straight up at the sound of her voice.

"Is she awake?"

The tech replied, "Is that you Mr. Ross? I had you in this room a few weeks ago. Is this your wife?"

He nodded yes, and she shook her head in disbelief.

"Honey, I have been right here since you had the surgery. You have hardly moved. They said you had to sleep off all the anesthesia. Brooke had to go home. She told me to come home and come back, but I wasn't going to leave you. I have been sitting here praying for us and for you to wake up. Thank you, Lord."

All I could do was breathe, listen, and purr.

The "Captain" came in and told me how well the surgery went. He said that he removed over sixty lymph nodes and sent them to the lab and that none of them showed any signs of cancer. I would be in the hospital a few more days and that I would be given another full body scan before being discharged. He wanted me to get out of the bed, sit up for a while, and try to walk to the bathroom.

The nurse came in and pulled the covers back. I had no idea I had a catheter and was using the bathroom through a tube. I had compression socks, and I was getting shots in my abdomen to keep blood clots from forming. There were tubes for everything. I looked like an octopus with tentacles moving in different directions.

The nurse began untethering me, but some of the tubes tangled beneath me, and I couldn't support my weight. Charles held me up and helped me to the chair. I looked out of the window and saw the beautiful autumn leaves on display. I pointed to them.

Charles said, "Once we get home, I'll go gather some and put them in a bowl in our room. Honey, did you hear what the Doctor said? He couldn't find any trace of cancer. Wait until I call Brooke, Staci, and your Dad and tell them."

Charles was on cloud nine. I was still crawling out of hell.

I sat up for a few minutes and walked to the bathroom. The nurse came to put me back on the bed and to hook up the feeding tube and monitor.

"Oh, by the way, Happy Anniversary." Charles reached under the bed and pulled out one red rose he bought at the hospital gift shop.

As he bent over to kiss me, Cancer appeared over his shoulder, "I'm not done with you yet."

I rolled over on the bed and mournfully purred until I fell asleep.

The following morning the "Captain" said, "It is time for the "big reveal." I am going to remove the bandages so that we could look at the external part of my handiwork."

He handed me a mirror, but I didn't want to use it. I would defer to the look in his and Charles' eyes as he unwrapped me like a mummy. When neither of them had an adverse reaction, I stole a quick peek in the mirror.

It was a long and deep scar that started beneath my right ear and circled to the front of my neck. I was being held together with staples of some kind. It reminded me of the old Frankenstein movie I had seen as a child. It wasn't as grotesque as I had imagined, but it was disfiguring. Part of me was gone. Cancer had claimed its pound of flesh. He said the staples would have to stay for another week and he would remove them in his office. I would be discharged from the hospital the next day to recover at home.

"Honey, it's not that bad. Remember those people you saw with major parts of their face or body missing? You know it could be worse."

I hadn't formed an opinion one way or the other. I was tired and in pain and wanted to go back to sleep and not think about it. Charles went for a walk. Once he was gone, I pulled the covers over my head.

I wanted to cry, but no tears would come. Instead, I grieved, dry-eyed, the loss of my body parts. It may not have looked bad, but every lymph node, muscle, nerve, skin, and drop of blood was mine. I had lost them to Cancer. I needed to mourn my losses, no matter who thought "it could be worse."

Stevie came to pick us up. He was solemn and still couldn't look at me. Brooke sent one of the beautiful scarves for me to wrap around my neck. With my head and neck covered, the only thing showing was my unhappy face. Charles sat in the front seat. I sat in the back looking at how the trees had shed so many of their leaves in the five days since my surgery. As we passed each tree and I saw my reflection in the car window, I thought of Charles' favorite Bible verse, Ecclesiastes 3:1-8.

> *To everything, there is a season*
> *A time for every purpose under heaven, a time to be born*
> *and a time to die*
> *A time to plant and a time to pluck what is planted*
> *A time to kill and a time to heal*
> *A time to break down, and a time to build up*
> *A time to weep, and a time to laugh*
> *A time to mourn, and a time to dance*
> *A time to cast away stones, and a time to gather stones*
> *A time to embrace, and a time to refrain from embracing*
> *A time to gain, and a time to lose*
> *A time to keep and a time to throw away*
> *A time to tear, and a time to sew*
> *A time to keep silent, and a time to speak*
> *A time to love and a time to hate*
> *A time of war, and a time of peace.*

In the last eight months, we had broken down, wept, mourned, cast away, lost, torn, kept silent, and been at war. Now, more than anything, we needed to heal, love and find peace.

THANKSGIVING

The week after I left the hospital, we learned that Charles was in remission. He was put on oral chemo with once a month blood transfusions and lumbar punctures. He was doing fantastic, and his doctor was proud of him. Brooke and Staci were happy that "Operation Save Papa Charles' Life" was successful.

My good news was my scans came back "Cancer free." Not cured, but "Cancer free." It was a major step forward in "Operation Save Mommy's Life." We celebrated our "Fraternal Twin" cancer free diagnoses.

The bad news was that I was not healing or getting stronger. I still could not eat or drink. I had severe mucositis because of the chemotherapy and radiation. Mucositis is the inflammation of the membranes in the digestive tract of the body from the mouth to the anus.

It was painful and felt like I was blowing my nose through my mouth. It would continuously form pools of mucous in the back of my throat that I couldn't swallow and needed to spit it out. I couldn't sleep for any period without having to get up to "blow my mouth." I was miserable, and if I thought projectile vomiting was terrible, this was a new low.

Brooke was starting to blossom. She and Stevie found out they were having a girl. They started thinking of names for our new princess. Despite my condition, Charles knew it was time for us to start looking for our own place. He felt strong enough to take care of me. We had been with Brooke and Stevie for seven months, and we needed to get out of the way for the newcomer.

We needed money. Charles applied for his Social Security before we left Arizona and he received a letter and check for nine months of payments in early November. It was like manna from heaven. We had enough money to open a bank account, buy a car, and a security deposit for an apartment.

Regenia called to check on us, and Charles told her our news and our plans. She said she had a nice car that we could buy. She and Jerry would bring it to us the following week.

* * *

They took the family out to dinner. The new baby was the talk of the evening, and Brooke's baby bump was now a round mound taking up space between her and the table. Regenia and Jerry once again came to our rescue. Though they drove their car home, I swear I saw one of Jerry's wings inching out under his jacket as he turned to leave.

Now we could find a place to live, but we couldn't decide whether to look near the hospital or close to Brooke. We opted to stay within a five-mile radius of Brooke. We had to call Bev and get our things out of her living room and on a truck to Atlanta. We wanted one bedroom, a small kitchen, one bath, no stairs, a laundry room, and access to a highway so that travel to and from the hospital would be easier. The hospital was a significant factor in our lifestyle—a year earlier, it wouldn't have appeared on our list.

* * *

Though I was languishing, I wanted to go to Cincinnati for Thanksgiving to see my Dad. Charles said he thought he was strong enough to drive the seven hours. It was still three weeks away, and I was hoping to be strong enough to take the ride.

We needed Georgia driver's licenses, registration, and insurance. As luck would have it, when we went to register the car, we got the same clerk that helped Debbie. She recognized me and apologized for her behavior that day. She said her aunt recently lost her battle with breast cancer and she was glad I was still fighting. I told her about Charles, and her eyes dropped. I saw the gruff civil servant attitude fade away.

The next Sunday, I went to church with Brooke and Bria. Everyone greeted me with an outpouring of love that made me cry tears of joy. I hadn't cried tears of joy for so long; it was a great release. As they fell into my mouth, I realized they tasted much different than the weighty, bitter tears of pain, anguish, frustration, and defeat. They were lighter, brighter, and sweeter. I needed more of them.

The sermon focused on gratitude and praising God, even through a storm.

Pastor Pollard referenced the book of Job— "Despite all of Job's financial losses, the loss of his children, the plague of diseases that overtook his body, the loss of his friends, the renunciations of his wife and the blaming him for his circumstances by some, he kept praising

127

God. He was grateful for each new day; even when each day brought more pain and suffering, he remained faithful." I believe Pastor Pollard knew I was coming and customized that message for me.

When the service was over, I stood in line to thank him. Before I could say a word, he wrapped me in a big hug. He said he knew how hard I was fighting and that one day I would have a remarkable testimony. When I heard him say those words, I cried more sweet tears. His beautiful wife hugged me. "That authority is looking good on you."

I replied, "I haven't been this uplifted and positive in a while. This church is a healing place."

As we turned to leave, another of Brooke's church members approached me, she mentioned that she moved into a newly constructed apartment complex and Brooke told her we were looking for housing. She suggested we give it a look. Charles was happy to see me smile and proposed that we drive by the apartment and go to the movies to give Brooke and her family some space.

* * *

Charles called Daddy and told him we were planning to come to Cincinnati for Thanksgiving. We were on speaker phone; Daddy and Mary were thrilled.

Mary asked "What special dishes do you want? I need to shop, cook, and have everything perfect for the feast."

When Charles told her his list, she asked, "What does Bari want?"

He told her I still couldn't swallow.

She sounded bewildered, "How can Bari be up to travel if she hasn't been able to eat in more than six months? I just can't imagine that, Charles."

He explained the feeding tube and the cans of sustenance, but I could still hear Mary's disbelief.

Daddy said nothing except, "Please bring her home safely to me, Sir Charles."

Charles replied, "Yes sir. I promise I will."

I love the relationship between Charles and my father. It is born of the respect and honor that they have for each other. The first time we visited Daddy, I could see them bonding over three Bs: baseball, bourbon, and Bari. I remember long ago trying to join them one Sunday afternoon—they laughed and went back to watching baseball, drinking bourbon, and ignoring Bari.

Thanksgiving arrived. As we prepared to leave, the weather took an ugly turn through the South and Midwest, mainly through Tennessee and Kentucky, which represented 85% of the drive to Cincinnati. Charles was willing to try because he gave Daddy his word, but Brooke firmly put her foot and protruding belly down, and that was the end of the conversation. Dad was disappointed but agreed that it was not safe.

I helped Brooke prepare a nice dinner with all the traditional foods and a few favorite desserts for Stevie and Bria. They were encouraging me to try a tablespoon of mashed potatoes or a spoon of Jell-O. I tried a spoon of potatoes, but it wouldn't go past my tongue. I made sure Kingston was included in the feast and discovered that, while he enjoyed the turkey and gravy, he loved cranberry sauce. Once he tasted it, when I gave him turkey, he would sit and look at it until I put cranberry sauce on it. He was spoiled, and I was thankful that he could enjoy the meal I couldn't.

Staci called from Houston, Texas. She was there to meet her "exclusive" man's family. I now knew his name was Christian. I'm sure she had told me before, but I couldn't recall. She sounded so happy and excited. I was grateful that she was enjoying herself and that life was moving forward for everyone. The new year was six weeks away, and I was looking forward to a calm end to 2009.

* * *

"The Captain" congratulated me on the progress I was making after the surgery. He removed the staples, and the scarring didn't look bad. In six weeks, I could begin physical therapy to help build up the muscles around my slumping right shoulder, which was throwing my posture and balance off.

I mentioned to him that my family was concerned about my inability to eat. He informed me that the swallowing muscles in my throat were atrophied for lack of use because of the radiation and I needed to see the swallowing therapist to strengthen the muscles. He went on to say it was common in patients who had head and neck cancer and part of the long recovery process.

* * *

We visited the apartment complex and it met our needs. We were ready to sign the lease and to move in January 9, 2010. We arranged for a truck to pick up our boxes from Bev in Phoenix and have them delivered to the apartment.

On December 8th, I developed hoarseness and a cough. I had an appointment the next day with my Rad-Onc. I mentioned it to him, he said it might be the mucositis. He recommended I drink warm salt-water to break it up and increase my water intake through the tube. I did that, but the coughing increased. Charles went to the pharmacy and bought some over the counter cough medicine and put it in the tube. I went to bed feeling something was wrong, but I didn't want to alarm anyone if, in fact, it was a simple cold.

At three o'clock in the morning, I asked Charles to take me to the emergency room. He was groggy and rolled over to go back to sleep. I pushed harder, and he snapped to attention.

"I don't know what's wrong with me, but I am sick, and I need to go to the hospital now!" I softly yelled.

As we were getting dressed Kingston started barking and Stevie came stumbling down the steps.

Charles said "Mommy is sick and wants to go to the emergency room. I will call when I know something."

There weren't many patients in the waiting area. The emergency room doctor had my information but admitted that she had to contact the oncologist on call. She would have to wait for instructions.

Within a few minutes, I was being wheeled down to radiology for a scan. I was no longer intimidated by the long tube or the sounds. They had become as routine to me as listening to the dishwasher.

My symptoms were vague. Besides a cough, I had feelings of malaise and foreboding throughout my body neither of which could be captured by a scan.

It was 5:30 a.m. when three handsome and healthy young men stepped around the curtain and strategically took their places around my bed.

The first one spoke with confidence, "Good morning Mrs. Ross. I am the Captain's Chief Resident, and these are my associates, who are also Residents."

They looked serious. The Chief Resident continued,

"We have looked at the tests and the scans and can find nothing wrong with you. We are going to discharge you from the emergency room and advise you to follow up with your next scheduled appointment."

I looked at Charles, and he seemed relieved that everything was fine and that we could leave.

As I lay there listening to the Chief Resident, I was also listening to "my body" telling me not to listen to him.

"Where is the Captain?"

"He is in surgery and won't be available until 5:00 p.m. this evening," he replied authoritatively.

"I'm not signing any papers until I see a doctor and while I respect the fact you are working on becoming doctors, if he is not available, I have two other doctors. Please call them over and please don't come back unless you are with the Captain," I said with exhausted conviction.

They stepped around the curtain and whispered to each other as they walked away.

Charles sat in the chair in disbelief.

"Honey, you sent those guys away. They can't find anything wrong with you. Maybe it's a cold. You aren't going to sign the papers if they bring them back?"

"Listen, they don't know me, all they did is read my chart, looked at some tests and decided to let me go home. I think my doctors know me by now, and might take a closer look and come to a different conclusion. I will wait here until 5:00 if necessary. I am sick, and I'm not leaving anytime soon. Please go get some breakfast and some fresh air."

Once Charles left, I laid back and listened to the sounds of the emergency room. They were different than the infusion center. They had a faster rhythm with nurses, techs, and staff race walking down the halls. I heard gurney wheels making sharp turns into the bays and carts being pushed behind them. There were cries of agony, cries of relief, and pleas for help. I heard young voices that had old pain and old voices that had new pains.

Suddenly I heard a familiar voice, and I looked over in the corner,

"I told you I wasn't through with you and I meant it," Cancer sneered as it slipped behind the curtain and blended in with the other sounds.

I rolled over and waited. I didn't know what I was waiting for, so I just waited. Sleep was not an option nor was being fed through the tube, not that I was hungry. The sense of being hungry had left me long ago, and while I understood I needed sustenance, I didn't have hunger pains or urges to ask for a feeding. So, I waited. Charles came back looking refreshed and told me he called Brooke to update her.

Around noon, my Rad-Onc came. He acknowledged Charles and congratulated him on being in remission.

He turned to me, "Mrs. Ross, I heard you gave the Residents a hard time this morning. We can't find anything in the tests. We obviously hear a cough and other than telling us you feel sick we don't have any reason to admit you to the hospital. We have no choice but to discharge you."

"It's the Cancer," I said.

"No, it's not. There is no sign of cancer since you had the surgery almost six weeks ago. All the tests are showing you to be cancer-free. I can't let you stay here."

I struggled to sit up in the bed and looked him in the eyes,

"We have been fighting this Cancer together for eight months. You know that I am not a hypochondriac nor do I make things up. I have trusted you and the rest of the wonderful team here that brought me this far. I need you to trust me now. I am sick. Maybe I have something that doesn't show up on the scans or the standard tests. Would you consider that? Please dig a little deeper. No one wants to go home more than me."

He patted me on the hand, "Okay, I'll be back."

Charles whispered, as I drifted off to sleep, "You gave him something to think about. Keep fighting!"

When I woke, The Captain and the Rad-Onc were at the foot of my bed. The Captain did not look pleased. I had been there more than twelve hours, and I was feeling worse; my cough was more intense, and my entire body ached. I was dizzy, and it hurt to talk. The Rad-Onc said he thought maybe I had cellulitis, which is a bacterial infection of the skin and is sometimes seen in surgical wounds.

I was pleased that he heard me and considered another possibility.

"We are going to admit you overnight for observation. Please promise me that if we don't find anything, you will sign the discharge papers tomorrow, Mrs. Ross."

"I'm not going to promise, but I will give it high consideration. Thank you so much for listening to me and looking past the tests," I squeezed his hand as he escorted me upstairs to a room.

It was 5:30 p.m. and we had been up since 3:00 a.m. Charles was exhausted. He took up his usual post on the recliner and fell asleep. After about two hours, he said he was going home to update Brooke and Stevie and to get his medications and he would come back. I begged him to stay home and get a decent night's sleep.

He said, "I'm not leaving your side. We are in this together. Besides, now that you are fighting, who's going to protect the doctors, residents, and nurses?"

My night nurse introduced himself; he was very Lincolnesque in stature. He was careful in every move he made and checked with me before and after he made any adjustments to the machines, my bed, or the lights. He took time to engage with me. I knew he was as busy as the other nurses, but he made me feel like I was his top priority. I will never forget him; another angel who entered my life and then flew away.

Charles returned around midnight. I was running a fever, had chills, and was shaking uncontrollably. I was nauseous, and my head ached down to the roots of my chattering teeth. The tech came for her routine vitals check and called the nurse. He assured me everything would be fine as he wrote on my charts. Charles kept adjusting the blankets around me and looked distressed.

In all my movements to get warm, I brushed my hand against my neck and then I felt it. I wasn't sure, so I let my fingers linger on it. When I was sure, I let out a roar that shook the entire room. A swelling was growing on my neck. When I showed it to Charles, he flung himself into the chair. The nurse came in with the head nurse. They were furiously taking notes and promised me the doctor on duty would be in to see me. I looked away from them with no energy to scream.

The doctor examined the area, ordered an antibiotic, and a sedative. As I was drifting off, I looked out the window and saw the shadow of Cancer, having visited other patients. It looked back at me with a smile on its face. I curled into fetal position and welcomed sleep.

The next morning, The Captain came into my room. I didn't know he was there until Charles shook me. I didn't want to open my eyes to let him or his words into my consciousness.

"Mrs. Ross, I have good and bad news for you,"

I didn't blink or speak. It was a very pathetic and familiar refrain.

He continued, "The good news is you don't have cancer. The bad news is you have an abscess in your neck that is infecting other areas. I am going to open it so it can drain it and treat you with strong antibiotics.

I will perform the procedure here in the room. You are going to be here for a while because these infections are very stubborn, and your immune system is not strong enough to help in the fight. Do you understand?"

I didn't understand.

Staci helped me understand; no matter what you call the medications, the opportunistic infections, the vomiting, the weight loss, the hair loss, the surgeries, the procedures, the setbacks or the grief, ultimately, "IT IS THE CANCER."

***

Charles seemed small in the chair. I could hardly see him, but I could hear him praying. The Captain was in the room, preparing me for the procedure. Before he started, he asked, "Would you mind if my

137

Residents come in and watch me? We are a University Hospital, and they are 'learning to become doctors.' as you reminded us yesterday. It's your right to say no, but it would be helpful."

I nodded okay; I realized that I had taught them all a valuable lesson about listening and trusting their patients, and that was not something they could get from the medical books or watching a surgical procedure. I wanted them to become the next "Captain of the Ship."

The Captain asked Charles to leave and made sure the area was sterile. The residents came in wearing gowns, masks, and gloves. The Captain talked through the entire procedure for the benefit of his students as they watched every movement of his steady and efficient hands. They stood at rapt attention as he spoke to them in a language that was unique to them and Greek to me. I laid there perfectly still daring to take the tiniest of breaths. I had the urge to cough and thought of the scalpel at my throat and suppressed it. In less than ten minutes, he was finished. Each of the residents thanked me for allowing them into my room again. When I looked, they were headed out to the Sea of Cancer with the Captain.

Charles went home to get things for the long haul. The more I tried to encourage him to stay to get some rest, the harder he resisted.

"Please don't ask me anymore. Things keep changing in a matter of minutes, and we need to hold on to each other for dear life."

After a few days, there was no improvement. The infection had spread. The Captain prescribed an additional antibiotic. I had nothing left. I no longer knew or cared about anything. I felt like I was slipping away. My body was of no use to me. It had been bombed and the only thing left was a shell.

I fell into a deep sleep, and my soul began to wander. Before I took flight, I needed to say goodbye and thank everyone close to me. In my unconscious, I called Brooke, Staci, Daddy, and Charles and told them I was ready to go, and I was at peace. I watched them cry as I floated away into a dark void. There was nothing, and I was nothing. I rested in nothingness, and it was good. Since there was no time and space, I don't know how long I was there, but my first recollection was of tiny pinpricks of light seeping through the darkness. I rested there and had no questions. Later, I heard small echoes of laughter coming from the lights. I enjoyed the sound. The light and laughter became more intense, and I was aware of a Presence. I rested there with the Presence.

Eventually, the Presence spoke to me, "What do you want to be now?"

I had no answer. It let me rest.

The Presence returned and asked again, "What do you want to be now?"

"I want to see my mother."

"You can't. She is no longer your mother. She is what she has chosen to be now."

"I don't know. What can I be?"

The Presence spoke softly, "The possibilities are infinite. Do you want to be a grain of sand? A color in a rainbow? A bird on the wing? A smile on a baby's face? A breeze over the ocean? A star in the sky?"

The Presence left. I rested.

When it returned, I said, "I am not finished being Bari."

When I woke up, Charles was standing over me praying and calling my name, "Bari, Bari."

ROLE REVERSAL

Charles said I was asleep and unaware for three days. After more than two weeks, I was discharged from the hospital— two days before Christmas. The Captain ordered a home health care nurse to follow up on the wound care. Charles asked him if I could travel by car to see my Dad for a few days. He said if Charles learned how to dress the wound, it would be fine. He prescribed a liquid antibiotic to go in the tube, gave us a mild sedative and wished us Merry Christmas.

When the nurse arrived, she showed Charles how to clean the wound and how to pack it to reduce the chance of infection. "Mr. Clean" nailed it on the first try. The nurse was impressed but ran him through the steps a few more times.

I slept while Charles packed our bags and got the car ready for the road. He went to the bank and withdrew traveling money and a generous gift for Brooke and Stevie. Brooke had doubts about my traveling so soon after being discharged from the hospital, but I told her I needed to see Daddy and she needed to be alone with her family for Christmas. She was blossoming with the new baby and in less than three months, she would be giving birth.

***

We left at midnight. Charles made sure to warm the car and have a few blankets to wrap me in for the trip. He was confident that by leaving at midnight, I would sleep for most of the trip and that we would arrive at Daddy's house for Christmas breakfast. He was a man on a mission.

Stevie helped me to the car and wrapped me in blankets like a newborn baby. It was dark and cold outside, but Charles had warmed the car, and it felt like an incubator.

I wanted to stay up to talk and keep him company as I did when we traveled. But this was nothing usual, and five miles later I was asleep. He stopped outside of Lexington, Kentucky to take a break. He woke me up, gave me a feeding and checked the bandage.

When we were about forty miles outside of Cincinnati, I tried to sit up for a few minutes. I couldn't. I caught a glimpse of the sun rising and I cried because I knew I was minutes from Daddy. I laid back and snuggled under the blankets.

We pulled up into his driveway as Mary opened the door. We stepped into the toasty house. There stood my eighty-six-year-old Dad. He took my arm, "Thank you, Sir Charles, I'll take care of her from here."

Charles said, "Yes, Sir," and took a step back.

Daddy led me down the steps to his "man cave" which he converted to a care center. He covered the couch with sheets and blankets. There was a roaring fire and he moved a table at the end of the couch to put any supplies needed nearby.

He still hadn't talked directly to me nor I to him for fear of us both breaking down in tears. In my fifty-seven years, I had never seen him cry. Each of his careful and deliberate movements said, "Baby, I love you, you are here, and you are safe. We don't need words or tears."

He sat in his recliner across from me without a word.

I listened to Charles and my stepmother upstairs talking as she prepared breakfast. I could hear the crackle of the new logs as Daddy added them to the fire. I could hear his sigh of relief as he tenderly pulled the covers up over my shoulders and brushed his hand softly against my cheek as I surrendered to sleep.

When I woke up, he was still sitting in his chair. My stepmother brought his breakfast on a tray, and the remnants of it were on the table next to him. Charles was upstairs in the bedroom resting from his heroic eight-hour drive. Dad helped me up from the couch, and Mary assisted me to the bathroom. When I came out, she asked if I wanted breakfast. I told her I still couldn't eat. I showed her the feeding tube.

I knew Charles was exhausted from the drive, but it was time for my feeding and wound care, and he was the only one who could do it. I waited another hour and reluctantly asked Mary to wake him. When he came downstairs with all the supplies, Daddy stoked the fire and went upstairs.

Charles said he and Daddy talked while I slept, and that Daddy had questions but didn't want to ask me. He suggested when I felt like talking, I should start the conversation. I told him Traci, Tim, and Arlene would be coming by later for dinner and we could have the conversation one time with everyone. He went back to bed, and Daddy came and put more logs on the fire and took up his post. As the flames jumped around in the fireplace, I saw Cancer peeking through the blaze. Daddy went over to the fire with the poker and stuck it in between the logs and Cancer disappeared up the flue with the smoke.

* * *

We hadn't seen Tim and Arlene since the illness invaded our lives, though they regularly called to check on us. My brother has always been the jokester of the family. I was prepared, and perhaps waiting, for him to find a bit of humor in making fun of my bald head or shrunken body. Instead, when he saw me, he grabbed me and broke down in tears. "Aww Sis, no baby, no!"

I couldn't make out the rest—it got swallowed by his tears.

Arlene first comforted him and said, "Tim, she, and Charlie are here and that's the most important thing."

When Traci arrived, she was jubilant. "Wow, Sis. The last time I saw you, I was worried. You didn't know I was there, as a matter of fact, you didn't know you were here. You're a little thin, but you've come a long way. Look at my brother Charles, you look amazing! So many people have been praying for you at my church."

Tim joined in, "Mine too."

Arlene refrained, "My church, my job, and my family."

Mary called us to the dinner table. She was a fantastic cook. Even her simpler meals went a few extra steps. On this day, she outdid herself. This meal was Thanksgiving, Easter, Fourth of July, and Christmas all prepared and presented at once. Charles and Tim had the biggest smiles on their faces. My Dad was looking at me, he was on guard for any misstep. Once everyone was served, he waited for Mary to make his plate and ate with his eyes never leaving me.

When Traci, Tim, and Arlene noticed that I didn't have a plate, they asked the obvious question. Charles told them I still had a feeding tube and couldn't swallow. I told them to enjoy their meal and that afterward I would tell them everything.

This was the opening Daddy was waiting for. He relaxed his guard a tiny bit and dived into his sumptuous meal with an eye on the three-layer chocolate cake.

After the meal, we gathered in the living room. Dad sat next to me on the love seat making sure there was a warm blanket around me. Charles and I relayed the story to them up to the minute that we arrived at the door. They were tearful, angry, amazed, and grateful as they rode the waves of the story.

My Dad held my hand, "I am proud of you and Charles. I ask the Great Master every day to bring you both through, and He has answered my prayers. Keep trusting and praying. You are stronger with two. NEVER give up. He will see you through, Cootsie."

When he called me "Cootsie," I burst into tears; nobody else on the planet is ever allowed to call me that but him. It is our unique bond and code.

Debbie called; she wanted to bring her parents to see us. Daddy was at the bottom of the stairs waiting to escort me to the toasty basement. He put chairs in place for Charles and Tim to watch the football game with him. He had the bourbon and eggnog set up on the bar. Charles couldn't have the bourbon but took a big glass of eggnog. Tim made a big glass of bourbon and skipped the eggnog. Dad had both and they toasted.

I laid there feeling so loved and blessed to have these three wise men caring for me on Christmas Day.

When I woke up, I heard Debbie's voice, "Where is she? Where is my Sister?"

Traci said, "She's downstairs with Daddy, Tim, and Charles. Give them a minute, and they'll be up."

It made me feel special that her father, Daddy Louis, who was not in good health, and Momma Ruth stopped by in the frigid weather to visit. I had last seen her mother at our wedding when she and my Dad took a turn on the dance floor.

When Daddy brought me, upstairs, Debbie jumped up and hugged me.

"Girl, I heard about the abscess from Brooke, and I started to come back down there, but she said there was nothing I could do so I stayed here and prayed."

146

Debbie's mother was a nurse for more than thirty years and kept her professional composure, but I could see the look of concern in her eyes. It was a look I had seen in the eyes of so many others over the past months.

Before she left, Debbie asked when we were going back home. Charles said Monday.

"Today is Friday. I hope you will be strong enough to go to church with me on Sunday."

Arlene spoke to me about caregiving for her mother who waged a fierce war against pancreatic cancer. She acknowledged Charles for fighting his cancer while caring for me. She said she was going to pray that I start eating. My brother didn't say anything and Traci gave me a hug.

Once they left, Daddy helped me upstairs to the door of the guest bedroom, and Charles walked me in. I was asleep before my head hit the pillow.

There were plenty of leftovers and Charles was in "food heaven." He couldn't stop eating, and Mary loves watching people enjoy her food as much as she likes preparing it.

"Help yourself, Sir Charles," Daddy said.

"Get some more, Charles," Mary encouraged him. He happily obliged them until he could hardly move.

True to her word, Debbie called to see if we were going to join her for church.

I told her, "We will come for a short while. If I get tired, we will leave."

* * *

When we arrived at The House of Joy, Debbie was waiting in the vestibule. As we entered the sanctuary, she danced all the way to her seat on the first row. The pastor's wife had an operatic soprano voice. She began singing, "Oh, Holy Night." Debbie fell on her knees upon the altar. There were tears and shouts from every pew as her voice climbed in a perfect crescendo. There were goosebumps over my body. It was my mother's favorite Christmas song, and I knew if she were here, she would have enjoyed the beauty of the moment.

The bishop stepped to the podium. He called us to the front of the church and introduced us as Debbie's friends, for whom the church was praying since May. He said we were survivors and the church erupted into thunderous applause. He asked me to give my testimony.

My neck was wrapped in a white bandage, I was very unsteady on my feet, but I thanked them for their prayers and told them I was released from the hospital a few days before and was grateful to share this moment with them.

When he gave Charles the microphone, he told them how he surrendered all to God after his diagnosis. The entire congregation was on their feet shouting, dancing, and praising. The musicians began playing "I Surrender All."

The pastor had his ministers make a circle around us. They anointed us with oil and prayed. It was an amazing feeling to be covered once again by so many anonymous angels. The prayers were healing and heartfelt, and I was warm from the top of my head to the bottom of my feet without needing a blanket. Charles and I were wrapped in prayer and were armored to move on to whatever was next.

We were jubilant when we arrive back at Daddy's house. He was concerned that we were out and about in the cold weather. He wanted one more evening to take care of me; the couch in the basement and the fire were ready.

Tim joined us for dinner and helped Dad with what remained of the Christmas bourbon. It felt good to hear Charles at ease and enjoying himself.

The next morning, Daddy said, "Sir Charles, keep the car warm and call us when you get home."

We waved good-bye, though snow was lightly falling, I felt so warm inside that I didn't think I would need the extra blankets I had used on the trip to Cincinnati.

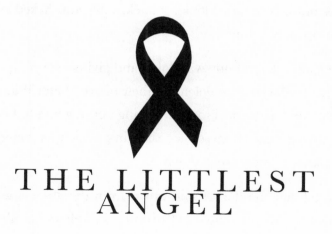

THE LITTLEST ANGEL

We returned to Atlanta happy and looking forward to a productive New Year. Our priority was moving into our apartment.

The next week, I had an appointment with the Captain. I wasn't feeling great, but I thought I was just still tired from the trip. However, the Captain let me know that my tiredness was a symptom of something much more serious.

"You have double pneumonia."

I looked at Charles; his head dropped so low all I could see was his ears. I heard what he said, and I believed what he said, but I had no reaction.

Charles asked him if I needed to go back to the hospital. He said I could be treated at home with more antibiotics. He thought the pneumonia was a residual of the abscess. I knew it was "Cancer " keeping me in its crosshairs.

I told Brooke I had pneumonia. She didn't say much, but the frustration showed on her face. I watched her shift her round belly and walk upstairs without looking back. Kingston licked my hand and went upstairs behind her.

I felt like a loser. Everybody was doing and giving everything, to help me, but the setbacks were defeating their efforts. Later that evening, Staci called and gave me a tongue lashing about going to Cincinnati and not taking care of myself, considering what was going on and how Brooke was being worn down.

I tried to tell her the doctor said it was from the abscess and never mentioned the trip, but she was frustrated as well and couldn't hear me.

The month-long treatments of antibiotics were wreaking havoc on my bowels. Though I wasn't eating, I was constipated and had thrush. I was in pain from my top to my bottom, but nothing hurt more than feeling I had used up my family.

Charles heard Staci's comments and said, "Honey, we are moving on January 10th. I will take care of everything."

*　*　*

Cancer stopped by to give me an update.

"I give you credit. You are a tough one. Every time I knock you down, you bounce back. I hadn't counted on the fortress of family and friends that would show up for you. As you can see from today's events, I am going to wear them down to nothing. They will turn on you and make it look like it's your fault. I win more than I lose and with each round, I learn more for the next one."

152

***

I had reached the depth of my lowest point with my daughters and it hurt.

Charles made the arrangements for our move. With the help of Stevie and one of his friends, we moved into our apartment on schedule.

As we were leaving, Brooke looked like a mother bird that teaches her babies to fly and then pushes them out of the nest to make room for the next brood. Kingston came and sat on my feet one more time. I gave him a belly rub and a big hug. Bria asked if we were going to be alright and Charles assured her that we would be fine and we would only be a few miles away.

The apartment was brand new. It was on the first floor of a three-story building. We had one bedroom, a small kitchen, and comfortable sized living room. The upstairs neighbor was quiet, but the neighbor across the hall played his music loudly. When Charles told him our situation, he was gracious and asked if he could help in any way; he lost his mother to cancer and was sympathetic.

The doctor said the pneumonia was clearing up and I was set for swallowing therapy. My right salivary gland was diminished and most of my taste buds were burned because of the radiation. Many foods, mainly bread and meat, would be difficult to swallow since there was not enough saliva to break them down and this would be permanent. I might never fully recover my ability to taste certain things the way I did before treatment.

153

I needed physical therapy to help build up the muscles in my chest and shoulder to support the areas where the surgeon removed tissue during the surgery.

I was ready. I wanted to help Brooke with the baby and to be a wife, not a patient.

My friend, Monica, told me her son, Coy, recently opened a physical therapy office. I've known him since he was in college. She said, "He will give you the "Family Discount," which meant it would be free.

I was near tears when I heard that. I was looking for a Physical Therapist, and I got another angel to help in the next step of my journey.

I told Brooke about Coy,

"I'll go with you to your first appointment. It will be good to see him again," she said.

We talked about how she was feeling, the nursery, and the upcoming Baby Shower. It felt good to talk about something positive and optimistic.

Coy greeted us with warm hugs. He had the prescription and the details of my surgery that related to my physical therapy needs. He'd taken the time to review the information thoroughly and created a rehabilitation plan that we would use for two months and then I could continue at home or the gym.

When I was finished, Brooke wanted to eat and asked if I would try ice cream. I put a spoonful on my tongue. It felt strange to have something in my mouth other than words, after ten months of being reliant on the feeding tube. It had no taste, not sweet, not milky, nothing. The only sensation was cold. I tried to let it sit on my tongue and drizzle down the back of my throat. It barely made it to the edge of my esophagus, and I gagged.

I was gagging so hard that tears came to my eyes. I left the table, went to the bathroom, and recovered my breathing. When I came back Brooke looked worried, "Are you okay, Mommy?"

"I'm fine. I guess if I'm going to try to eat, I should do it at home."

When we got in the car, she said, "I'm glad you tried."

"Next stop, swallowing therapy." I believed that it was going to be harder than the physical therapy.

***

The esophagus is one of the most active muscles in the body. It maintains its strength through use. Since I had not used mine for months, it had weakened and atrophied, much like a broken leg in a cast. When the cast is removed, the leg looks shrunken and shriveled and may not be able to support your weight. The base of my tongue and esophagus were shriveled and weakened.

Over the next month, I was given a series of exercises and tests to begin strengthening and building up the muscles that allowed me to swallow. At the end of four weeks, I could drink liquids from a straw and eat very soft foods. I felt confident enough to make an appointment to have the feeding tube removed. At the end of eight weeks, I could lift my arm and was able to lift eight pounds of weight.

This feat was right on time because Brooke was days away from delivering a seven-pound baby girl.

I focused on the arrival of the new baby. I wanted to see her little face and look into her eyes.

I wanted to shop for a few things, but they received many gifts at the baby shower, including duplicates there was nothing left for me to buy. I gave them a certificate for on-demand babysitting with three-days prior notice. They knew Charles and I would babysit at the drop of a hat if asked.

On March 26, at 3:30 a.m., the phone rang, "Mommy, my water broke. We are on our way to the hospital."

"Okay, I'll come to the hospital around ten a.m., maybe by that time you'll be close to delivery."

I dozed off, the phone rang again,

"She's here," Stevie said. "She arrived at 6:26 a.m. and she is 7½ pounds, healthy, and beautiful," he gushed.

"How is Brooke?" I asked.

"Do you want to talk to her?"

"No, tell her I'm on my way."

I pushed hard on Charles to wake him and tell him the news.

"We have to get to the hospital. I have to see her and hold her as soon as possible."

I jumped in the shower and let the water cover me from head to toe. I closed my eyes and touched every part of my body that was ravaged.

As I stepped out of the shower and looked in the mirror, I noticed my hair sprouting little curls, and my burns and surgical scars were healing. My ability to eat by mouth was improving and I was getting stronger. I dressed and paced the floor while waiting for Charles, trying to imagine who the baby looked like. I wanted to count her fingers, toes and kiss her cheeks.

The hospital was forty-five minutes away. When we got there, Stevie was lying on the couch with the baby on his chest. Brooke was in bed smiling and assured us that she and the baby were fine. Charles said we should pray and give thanks for the new life. I sat down and watched Stevie bonding with the baby and caught quick peeks of her under the blanket.

I asked to hold her, and Stevie placed her in my arms. She was alert. I looked into her big brown eyes. I kissed her baby toes and fingers. I smelled her baby breath. I tenderly ran my hand over her baby hair. It was love at first sight. I was concerned that she was at the edge of my weight limit, but Stevie stayed there. My arm gave out sooner than I had hoped for, so I gave her back.

Charles was reluctant to hold her. "She's tiny. I'm scared I might drop her, or she might slip out of my arms." But he couldn't resist, so Stevie laid her in his arms.

The nurse came in and gave Charles a pink pin that said, "I AM THE NEW GRANDFATHER." I couldn't stop looking at her and thinking here is a little cherub angel sent to help us joyfully move on.

157

* * *

On the way home, we stopped to check on Bria. She was just getting home from school, and we were able to show her pictures of the baby. We also had a blanket that they wrapped the baby in, and we gave it to her so she could use it to play with Kingston so he would recognize the smell of the baby.

Kingston was happy to see us, and he almost knocked me down with his show of affection. I was glad to see him. We played with him for a while, and when we got ready to go, he happily walked us to the door. I knew once he smelled the baby's blanket, his new job was going to be protecting her. He sensed that his assignment was over with us and he knew we loved him.

I called Daddy to tell him and Mary about the new baby. Dad joked that he had so many grand and great-grandchildren that he had lost count. He would call her "Skylark," because they represent joy.

Two days later, they came home. We went over to visit and saw that Kingston was anxious about the new baby. He was barking, jumping, and wagging his tail. Stevie gave him another blanket, and once he recognized the smell, he calmed down. Charles and I brought a homemade dinner and I held our littlest angel.

158

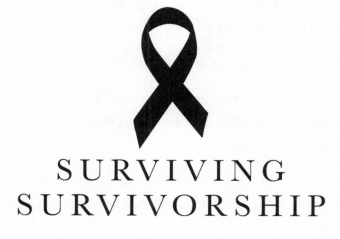

SURVIVING SURVIVORSHIP

Things finally calmed down. Our doctors gave us three rules: eat healthy, exercise, and avoid stress. While the first two were a matter of choice and discipline, the third involved outside forces that weren't under our control.

One morning at four o'clock, I woke up to a noise that I recognized. It was Charles in the living room muffling his cries. As I moved the few steps toward the door, my mind started racing in different directions, none of them positive. Before opening the door, I filled my lungs with two deep breaths. After all we had been through, I couldn't imagine what news was waiting for me on the other side. I said a prayer and turned the knob.

Charles was sitting in the dark, so I didn't turn on the light. When I came into the room he didn't move, nor did he stop crying.

I sat down next to him and waited for him to speak. All my thoughts were very dark: sickness, cancer, and death—I didn't say a word.

He cried for another few minutes, "Why haven't my children called or contacted me?" he wailed.

I didn't know what to say or how to feel.

Charles sniffled, trying to reign in his tears. "I guess I have to move forward. The doctor said don't stress, but this has me upset, and I've been thinking about it for a while."

In the last year, Charles had battled his cancer. He had taken care of me through my battle, setbacks, and challenges. But through it all, he hadn't had a chance to count his sorrows and grieve his losses. There was absolutely nothing I could say or do. I tried reaching out to them earlier in our journey, and their rebuff was swift and certain.

Charles needed time to grieve before he could enter his "new normal." We were both struggling with Post Traumatic Stress Disorder (PTSD), and other things were going to surface that we hadn't recognized or dealt with while we were actively at war with Cancer.

I grew concerned that Charles was becoming depressed and suffering from Chemo-Brain. Since we both had Chemo-Brain sometimes, we would laugh when we couldn't remember something and other times it would lead to arguments and harsh words. The mood swings became unpredictable, and sometimes, we went days barely speaking to avoid an argument.

One evening, Charles went to meet one of his nephews who was passing through Atlanta. On the way home, Charles hit a car. When he called me, the young man he ran into was threatening him, and he was in the car with the doors locked waiting for the police. I asked

Stevie to go over to check on him. When he got there, the police officer was finishing the report.

When Stevie called to update me, he said, "Papa Charles hit his head and I'm taking him to the emergency room. He seems confused and may have a concussion."

At 2:00 a.m., Stevie called. He left Charles because he had to go to work.

Cancer tried to whisper in my ear, but I wouldn't let it. Though each minute seemed like an hour, I stayed focused and waited until I could hear all the facts.

At 6:30 a.m., Charles walked through our door. He looked bedraggled, but he said the news was good, and there was no sign of a concussion. He didn't think the damage was bad, and it could be fixed in a week. I suggested that we get some sleep and discuss the accident later.

The next morning, he picked up a rental car and we went to meet the insurance adjuster. When I looked at the car, my heart dropped.

Before I could speak, the adjustor said, "It's totaled."

"Do you know what that means?" he asked when we didn't respond.

"It means we don't have a car. The only insurance we could get was liability because of the age and mileage," I fumed.

"Honey calm down. We will figure something out. It didn't look so bad last night, but it was dark, and I was confused."

Two days later, we saw an ad for a used car that we could afford.

161

When we got to the used car lot, the car from the ad had been sold. The salesman had another car he thought we might be interested in, but, of course, that car was more money than the one we originally set out to spend.

"Charles, this feels like a bait and switch." I said, not fooled one bit by the salesman's tactics.

They ignored me and continued to negotiate. I went to the restroom. When I came out, the salesman directed me to an office where Charles was sitting with the "Closer" going over financing and terms.

When he asked me if there were any questions, I shook my head, knowing that if I spoke, I would explode. I decided my only choice was not to sign any papers or participate in what would be his choice and his alone. Because of his low credit score, the interest was bordering on loan shark rates.

When we walked out, Charles was the owner of the bait and switch car, and I was the owner of a major headache and foul mood. We argued all the way home and then didn't talk the rest of the day. Suddenly, it felt like we weren't playing on the same team anymore. It was more "every man for himself and God for us all."

Every time we tried to have a conversation, it seemed to devolve into an argument or blame game. We began to withdraw and avoid each other, which was hard to do in a one-bedroom apartment.

It was evident that we were struggling with our new normal. It was also painfully obvious that we didn't know what to do about it. We didn't have a road map or GPS for new normal, and it was increasingly apparent that it looked different to each of us.

Charles would bring up what we lost in Phoenix, and I would say, "Why are you talking about that? It's over and we have to concentrate on our health and future."

He said that he would talk about it and I couldn't stop him. When he brought it up, I would leave the room or turn up the television.

He needed to find someone to talk to about his losses, his children not being there for him, and his future.

I couldn't be that person.

Most important to me was to answer the question, "What do you want to be now?" The past was the past, and I needed to move forward not look back. After a month of mutual alienation, I was at a doctor's appointment and picked up a brochure from Winship about a Survivorship Program to assist post-treatment cancer patients in transition to their new normal, both physically and emotionally. I made separate appointments for us. Once again, our "fraternal twin" cancers caused us to have similar but different needs; we were both struggling in our own unique ways. I thought maybe at some point we may need to have joint counseling, but for now we needed to address our individual concerns with the Program Director.

I received an extensive questionnaire and a brief letter explaining the goals of the program. The meeting with the Program Director was scheduled to last two hours. I was impressed she could be thorough and address my concerns. I did my homework and organized my questions before the meeting.

163

I knew I was in the presence of an angel.

Joan was welcoming, knowledgeable about my medical history and compassionate. She allowed me to lead the meeting with questions about my treatment. She said late-stage Head and Neck cancers have one of the most difficult treatment programs and they have a significant rate of recurrence.

The Captain had told me that early in my treatment, but my focus was on remission not on recurrence. Now that she brought it to my attention, I needed to think about what I could do, if anything, to keep it from returning. She gave me a sly nod for not leaving the emergency room and demanding another look.

I told her about the relationship problems Charles and I were having, and she wasn't surprised. She admitted she had never worked with nor heard of a couple who had cancer at the same time. She worked with cancer patients for over twenty-five years, and we were her first. She couldn't discuss Charles' medical records or treatments with me but assured me we were still afflicted with "chemo brain," and some of the emotional upsets and challenges were directly related to that.

She suggested we remain patient and give each other space to grieve and renew at our own pace. It was sad that Charles' children weren't there for him. In her years of practice, she saw it many times; some of the closest family members turn their backs on patients and that, while it hurts, you must press forward. She gave me a referral to a marriage therapist but suggested I wait until after she met with Charles before making an appointment.

Charles did not go to his Survivorship appointment until three months later. Joan told him that with his cancer, there was a significant rate of relapse. She suggested we take day trips together but to also find an interest that he liked to do by himself or with male friends. Her experience told her that whatever was going on with his children was probably happening before the cancer showed up.

We found a book on day hikes in Georgia. Since it was late summer and humid in the Atlanta area, we went north to the mountains where the weather was cooler and the views spectacular. I found a book club that met once a month. Charles found a fishing buddy. We were mindful of our tenuous health status, but we were making progress and moving forward, one day at a time.

Our one-year anniversary of being cancer free was coming up. We were during planning a small celebration when Charles developed a cough. The doctor said it was bronchitis.

He took medicine for a few days, said he felt better, and was going to make a trip to see his daughter in Maryland. I was stunned he would drive for fourteen hours by himself. I didn't understand why he was risking his health to travel to see her.

He stayed for a week. I refused to take any calls from him while he was there. When he got home, he stumbled through the door. It was apparent he was sick with a fever, chills, and a worsening cough.

The next morning, he was listless. I called his doctor, and she told me to bring him to her office.

The bronchitis developed into pneumonia. His blood count dropped, and he needed a blood transfusion. The waiting room, despite the crowd, was eerily quiet. I found a single chair in a far corner and picked up a magazine. I heard someone call my name. I turned thinking it was a nurse but because they said "Bari" and not Mrs. Ross, I thought it was someone who knew me.

I looked through the crowd but didn't recognize anyone, and when I looked behind me, I saw Cancer. It had a smug look. "Low blood count, infection, blood transfusions. I'm back for Charles."

I put the magazine down and looked around the room at the patients in various stages of battling blood cancers. I asked myself why we were back here now, after months of being away.

I wanted to blame Charles for driving fourteen hours each way, for doing whatever he did while he was away trying to start a new normal. I knew Cancer was right; there was nothing I could do if he relapsed. Anger was not the answer, and neither was blame. I closed my eyes and said a prayer When I opened my eyes, I saw Cancer move on, taunting and haunting other families.

***

Skyelar was in daycare and I missed her. Because Charles was sick, I thought it was best that we stay away until he got well. With his weak immune system, I didn't want Charles to be exposed to anything the baby might pick up at the center. We could not afford for his condition to get any worse.

166

Charles' bout with pneumonia lasted for six weeks. I was exhausted and concerned about my health, but I knew we couldn't go back to the people we relied on before. No host of angels was going to descend to help. No matter what direction this was going, it was up to Charles and Bari to get through it.

The pneumonia cleared up, and the doctor scheduled a blood transfusion in mid-December with the hope of jump-starting his immune system to avoid a relapse. She also changed his medications and chemotherapy regimen. The holidays were uneventful, the one bright spot was watching Skye enjoying the lights and Kingston following her as she took her first steps.

In January, we got good news. Charles' blood counts were improving, and his lungs were clear. It seemed as if his immune system was strengthened. We were hibernating, only going out when necessary and trying to avoid anything perceived as a health risk which turned out to be everything except sleeping and eating. No friends, no book club, no day trips, no fun, and no life.

March went out like a lion, but the lion stayed through April. Every time Spring tried to escape from Winter, it was pummeled by cold wind and rain.

I thought we would be out and about by Easter, but Easter wasn't until late April, and the weather was still crisp and cool. We were in a holding pattern. Like the buds on the trees or the petals on the flowers, we wanted to burst through and thrive, but every time we tried, a storm came and pushed us underground.

In mid-May, the sun and heat broke through. The temperatures were consistently rising, and so were our hopes.

* * *

After Charles' blood count numbers stabilized, he found a park nearby with beautiful hiking trails. The park has a reflecting pond in its center, full of ducks and geese. We enjoyed feeding the ducks and walking the trails. It was therapeutic and helpful as we once again attempted to move forward.

Charles started going back to the gym on a regular basis, and I joined him. We started out in a class called Silver Sneakers. It was for seniors and people who hadn't been active in years. Some of the participants were elderly, others were recovering from recent operations, some had chronic diseases, and at least two of us were recovering from cancer. Many of the participants remained seated doing their exercises in their chairs the entire class. Some people did half the class seated, and the other half was standing. Only a few people could do the whole class standing.

What impressed me was the instructor. Her name was Amy. Her disposition and attitude with the group were warm and enthusiastic. She would show us an exercise and how it could work whether seated or standing.

I liked when she said, "Do what you can! Forget about the rest."

She gently nudged us to continue and not give up. She explained the benefit of each exercise and gave us healthy eating tips.

I started a spin class that was taught by a retired Army Colonel named Steve, and he yelled and screamed at the class like we were on a mission to save our other riders. I loved it and bought the whole "no pain no gain" theory of working out. Though I had suffered plenty of pain, I thought this was good pain, At the end of each day, I fell into the bed exhausted and barely able to move but self-assured that we were doing what we needed to do to fight a recurrence.

We became fanatic about exercise, food, and water. Every meal, drink, and cleaning agent choice became suspect. New words crept into our vocabulary—organic, GMO, gluten free, dairy free, sugarless, sugar free, low sodium, no sodium, soy milk, almond milk, coconut milk, spring water, purified water, smart water, vegan, vegetarian, farm fresh, farm raised, caged, free ranged, grass fed, grain fed, caffeine free, decaffeinated, vegetable oil, olive oil, coconut oil, herbal, fresh, probiotics, prebiotics, antibiotic free, fragrance-free and chlorine-free.

It was new, but it was not normal. It was evident that establishing a new normal was not easy and that we tended to go to the extreme. We backed off furiously exercising six days a week. I settled on going to a yoga class twice a week and alternating between walking and spin classes for cardio.

Charles' doctor invited him to join her in a 10k run for Leukemia. He came in third place in his age group. His doctor was very proud of him and suggested that he continue to run as part of his recovery. He joined the Atlanta Track Club and won several ribbons in his age group. I walked and collected participation tee-shirts.

Our greatest joy was babysitting. Skye was walking and very active. Keeping her was a real work out. We did cardio running after her and her curiosity. We lifted weights picking her up and carrying her through the store. We did yoga assuming various positions on the floor playing Legos or reading to her. We ate healthy carrots, apples, bananas, and green beans. We drank healthy juices and plant-based milk. We loved her, and she loved us. Doing this felt like a new normal that we could live with and enjoy. Watching her grow was giving us new life. She was our youngest angel and lifted us up to new heights with her learning to say a new word every day, learning to climb stairs or trying to ride Kingston like a pony.

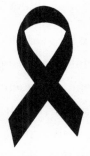

TO FORGIVE
OR NOT FORGIVE

Stevie was over the moon in love with Skye. Sometimes when he came to drop her off, he wouldn't leave. One day, he asked me where Charles' children were. He said he couldn't believe that after two years they had not come to Atlanta to see us nor had they said thank you to anyone for standing in the gap for them. Over the years I had known Stevie, I had never heard him say a harsh word about anyone. All I could tell him was,

"Son, I don't know why, and I don't have an answer from them."

I didn't want to be angry or stressed out, but it was always the elephant in the room during interactions with family and friends. Charles' sister, Polly, arranged a family "Lovefest" party for us at her home in Virginia; it was a celebration of our survival. Charles and I were excited to see the many family and friends who helped us. I thought this might be an opportunity for Charles to speak to his daughter or son and clear the air. Neither of them came nor did they send a card or call. I felt sorry for Charles, and I determined that it was the end of my having any expectation that things would improve.

I called my one reliable source for guidance. I told Dad my experience with the puzzle of Charles' children during our darkest days and how my feelings of disappointment and resentment would flare up from time to time. He said there were two choices: I could forgive them and move on, or I could let their actions or lack of action interfere with my progress. I asked him how to forgive when I don't trust.

"Cootsie, the prayer is to forgive, it says nothing about trust. Trust has to be earned forgiveness is a gift you give yourself."

I knew he had an answer for me that would help clear up my emotional fog. Forgiveness was on the menu. Trust was not.

In October, we traveled to Ohio to celebrate my Dad's eighty-eighth birthday. I was able to get tickets in a suite on the fifty-yard line to see a Bengals football game. He was sitting in his big brown recliner when I told him about the plans, and he made excuses why he didn't want to go. I was confused because I knew he was a fan.

I pressed him on why he didn't want to go.

"I don't like the quarterback, I don't like the coach, the parking is terrible, it will be cold," he said.

He stood up to walk up the stairs to get a beer. I watched as he stumbled a bit before gaining his balance. I sat still and waited for him to come back.

When he sat down, I answered all his objections,

"Daddy, you still like football, so we can go for the love of the game

172

and not root for the Bengals. We've got VIP parking, so we are right next to the stadium. Our seats are in a temperature-controlled suite, and the temperature on Sunday is forecast to be seventy-five degrees and sunny."

I kept my eye on him as he moved about and noticed he was starting to take little shuffle steps. Later that night, when he and Charles went to bed, I asked Mary about his health. She said he had been to the doctor and had gotten a good report, but he was starting to lose his balance and stumble and fall on occasion.

Sunday morning at 7:30, Dad was sitting on the couch dressed in his Bengals regalia. I hugged him and smiled. Charles told him he had a surprise when we got to the park. Traci, Tim, and his son TJ were going. The weather was perfect. When we got to the lot, TJ let down the back door, and Charles set up a tailgate party replete with a long submarine sandwich, salads, chicken wings, a cooler of beer, wine and soda, fruits and a birthday cake. To top it off, we had stopped on the way from Atlanta through the Bourbon Trail in Kentucky and bought his favorite brand.

* * *

We headed toward the suite, Dad couldn't keep the pace and was struggling to walk. I asked him if he wanted Tim to get a wheelchair. He declined. Charles met us with a wheelchair and a transport agent to push it. He offered it to Daddy and once again the answer was no. Charles used it and when we got to the suite Charles was sitting in his seat having a beer and holding one in his hand for Daddy.

Though we had eaten at the tailgate, the suite came with a full complement of food, drinks, and a waiter. The seats were perfect, and TJ who played football from his childhood through college was our ideal play by play man. Daddy was in seventh heaven with his son, grandson, son-in-law, and daughters watching his favorite sport with him.

The Bengals lost, but it did not diminish the significance of the day. When the game was over, I had two wheelchairs waiting outside the door of the suite one for Daddy who sat in it immediately and one for Charles, who didn't need it but used it to keep Daddy company. As we drove back to the house, I listened to Daddy and the men go over every play and referee call as if they each had the same camera in their heads and had recorded it from the same angle. I was amazed at how much Dad could remember, to the smallest detail, and how his sons were reveling his knowledge of the game.

Mary had a full dinner ready and another birthday cake waiting. Debbie came over, and Daddy was pleased to see her, "How's my other daughter, why didn't you come to the game with us?"

"Daddy Herman, you know I don't follow sports, but I came this evening to celebrate with you" she replied.

"Well you should have come for the fun, the food and the family time," he smiled and winked at me.

After dinner as he got up from the table, Daddy stumbled and almost fell, but Tim moved quickly and caught him before he hit the floor.

"Are you alright, Daddy?" Traci asked.

"Don't worry; I'm tired it's been a long day. Thank you all. I had a

174

great time, and this has been one of the best birthdays I've had in eighty-eight years. I'm going to bed now," he said as he headed for the stairs with Tim, Charles, and Mary behind him.

Early the next morning, Mary made us breakfast and said Dad wanted us to come to his room before we left. I wanted a few minutes alone with him.

He was very upbeat. I walked over and gave him a hug and told him how proud I was of him and how much I loved him. He was proud of us and how hard we fought and how far we had come. He never imagined being in the stadium and a private suite and I had spoiled him. We knew that this was another one of our special Daddy and daughter moments and were at peace with whatever the future may hold. When Charles came in, he shook his hand, "Whatever you do, you take care of my daughter."

We got in the car, I kept looking at the door to see Daddy and Mary waving and saying, "goodbye, drive safely, call us when you get home" at least five times. I saw Mary, small and tired, wave twice and close the door.

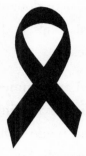

THE UNRELENTING SPECTER

It was time for more doctor appointments. I had my annual physical and mammogram and Charles his physical and colonoscopy. We also had our cancer-related scans. We were in a very good place health wise and were doing everything the doctors prescribed.

I started to put on weight, and though my taste buds were not fully recovered, I was finding things to eat that were healthy and satisfying. Soups were a big part of my diet, and I learned to add herbs and spices to give them variety. I fell in love with Vietnamese Pho, a dish full of vegetables and noodles in a tasty broth. Many of the things I enjoyed before were now unwelcome in my diet, some because of taste others because of texture. My taste buds were at fifty percent of their function, so many things like fresh fruit and salad greens tasted metallic. Juices were bitter and burned when I swallowed them due to their acidity. All meat was out due to its texture and flavor. Because of the lack of saliva to break it down when I chewed it, it became impossible to swallow. Chocolate was bitter and biting; bread was out

177

because it turned into a big ball of dough that wouldn't break down. I found seafood, eggs, oatmeal, soups, and cooked vegetables to be the most comfortable things to eat.

A few days after our annual appointments, we got results from our respective doctors. Charles was holding his paperwork up like a student who learned he had made honor roll. He was happy and beaming like a hundred-watt light bulb. He didn't notice that I was sitting on the couch looking at my report with disbelief. When he did, he ran over to my side.

"What's wrong, Honey?" he said as the smile that was on his face collapsed into a frown from the corners of his eyes to the curl of his lips. I handed him the papers to read, but he pushed them back towards me. "Please, just tell me. I don't want to read. Talk to me."

"The mammogram report says they see something suspicious in my right breast and that I need to come in for further test and a possible biopsy."

I didn't hear his reaction. In the glass frame over his shoulder, I was staring Cancer in the eye and it glared back with a sly grin.

A week later, I was in the breast imagining clinic. I wasn't hysterical or sad; I was angry. When I sat down with the doctor, before he could explain the mammogram reading, I attacked him with a barrage of questions.

"I have had multiple full-body scans in the last three years and a mammogram last year. How could anything have been missed? Does it look like a tumor? How big? How long has it been there? What are we going to do about it? When are we going to begin treatment? Chemo, radiation, surgery, or all of them? Will I lose my hair again?" I railed at him.

It felt like Deja' Vu all over again.

"Hold on, Mrs. Ross. Please calm down and allow me to explain where we are," he said calmly.

I took a deep breath to steel myself against his words. He couldn't understand the ongoing adversarial relationship that Cancer and I had and that this felt like another sneak attack. I was practicing the "Art of War" rule number one: "Know your enemy," and he was practicing medicine. I knew my enemy, and I knew every minute I waited, Cancer was gaining ground.

He turned on a screen that showed my mammogram.

"First let's look at the left breast. See how clear and consistent the picture looks? Now look at the right breast. See the shadow and the dark area. That area is what needs further investigation. Today we are going to take some higher resolution pictures to see if we can determine what this is. Once we get these back, we will meet again and talk about next steps. I know you had a battle with cancer and are still recovering, which is why we are more concerned than usual. Please don't jump to conclusions."

* * *

Outside of Winship is a space called the Healing Garden with a beautiful fountain surrounded by seasonal plants and shade trees. I found a bench and sat under a Japanese Maple tree. I closed my eyes and prayed.

Everything around me was quiet, despite the cars going by and the people in conversation nearby. I couldn't hear anything but silence. As I started to leave, a small whisper made its way to my consciousness.

"What do you want to be now?"

I sat back down and made a mental list. I want to be strong; I want to be wise; I want to be cancer-free; and I want to be Bari.

Brooke called to see what happened at the appointment.

"Mommy, don't get too upset. They have got to take their time and be very thorough to make sure they don't miss anything."

As I hung up the phone, Charles came home.

"How did it go with the doctor?"

I told him about the time I spent in the Healing Garden and that I had decided to go through the process suggested by the doctor before thinking the worst. I requested that he do the same thing. He seemed relieved and we made a toast with a glass of freshly brewed tea.

That night after Charles went to bed, I looked on the internet for information about breast cancer. I had learned quite a bit about our "Fraternal Twin" cancers. I knew nothing about breast cancer. I was up most of the night looking at the different types of breast cancers, the various treatments, the side effects of the treatments, and the survival rates. I read for education and information. I tried hard not to say, "Yes, that's me" when I read a statistic or profile that fit me like a customized radiation mask. I tried harder not to touch the scar on my neck as I looked at pictures of women with scars where their

180

breasts once proudly protruded. I tried hard not to fall into despair when I read the number of deaths for women with breast cancer, only exceeded by the number who die from lung cancer.

No matter how hard I tried not to think about it, it crept into my mind. I started noticing women with bald heads, women with orange colored skin, pink ribbons, car decals with references to tatas or boobies, "Race for the Cure" promos, and paraphernalia in stores from tee shirts to coffee mugs. I had seen it all many times before, but now it was personal. In the shower, I would feel for a lump; there was none. I would look in the mirror and could see nothing unusual about the shape or coloration. I was regularly checking my phone, mailbox, and email for information from the doctor, all while trying to hide my anxiety from Charles.

I finally received a call from the Breast Clinic asking me to schedule an appointment to review the results. I asked for the next available date and couldn't get in within a week. I assumed that if it was as bad as I thought they would have called me sooner. I was tired, and it was getting impossible to hide my concerns from Brooke and Charles. I wanted to call Staci and talk to her about my feelings, but she was now happily engaged and making wedding plans, and I didn't want to intrude into that space.

I walked into the appointment calm but skeptical. I was ready to listen and learn. The doctor got straight to the point, "We still aren't sure what we are looking at, and we have to do a biopsy to determine what it is. It is a simple procedure where we insert a needle and extract some tissue. I know you are familiar with this. The good news is we can do it here in the clinic and will have results in three days."

181

Christmas was less than a month away. I got Skye to lift my spirits. Charles and I took her to the mall to see the holiday decorations. She was twenty months old, running everywhere, and saying quite a few words—especially "no." She was a delight, making funny faces and manipulating Charles to do her bidding. I bought her several books and attempted to read them to her, but she wanted to read them to me, so I surrendered to "See doggie, see apple, see horsey, see nabana." I couldn't help but laugh. A day with her was just what I needed to feel joyful.

Charles was very talkative on our way to the clinic. He wanted to plan a midwinter cruise. I listened but didn't say much; I wanted to get some answers before I started making any plans.

When we arrived for my appointment, Charles wanted to sit in the general waiting area, not in the Breast Clinic Area with the women. The nurse led me to a locker room to put on a gown. She reached into a warmer and handed me a soothing robe which helped calm me. She then directed me to a second waiting room. The room was eerily quiet. Many of the women had buried their faces in magazines; some were texting or surfing on their cell phones.

I said, "good morning" when I entered the room; only one woman responded, and it was a muffled "morning." I guess there was nothing good about it since we were all sitting here waiting for the various tests that may or may not bring good news.

My nurse escorted me to the procedure room. She numbed my breast and then the doctor and his assistant came in to perform the needle biopsy.

In less than five minutes it was over, and he said he would have results in three days. He stepped out, and his assistant put a band-aid over the area. I was instructed to keep the area clean and take over the counter medicine if I experienced any pain.

As I changed clothes and took a quick peek in the mirror, I couldn't see anything because of the band-aids, and I couldn't feel anything because it was numb. I went to the lobby to look for Charles, but he wasn't there. He was having a snack in the cafeteria. I told him not to hurry; I would sit in the area and listen to the piano player.

A man who checked us into the infusion center saw me and called out, "Mrs. Ross, what are you doing here? I thought you were through with treatment."

I told him I was there for a follow-up visit without going into any detail. He then looked at me very sheepishly and asked in hushed tones, "How is Mr. Ross?"

I answered, "Turn around and ask him for yourself. He's coming through the door."

I heard him exhale as he turned to greet Charles.

He laughed heartily, "You guys have made my day, to see both of you doing well is a miracle. I want to wish you the best for the holidays. God bless you."

Charles and I turned to leave the building, and we ran into his doctor who was getting off the elevator. "Mr. Ross, good to see you and Mrs. Ross."

She wished us a Happy Holiday and sped off to assume her position in the ranks of the battalion of doctors fighting cancer at the center.

I said to Charles, "Let's get out of here. It's starting to feel like a reunion."

We drove past an Indian restaurant near the hospital that we enjoyed and decided to stop there for a late lunch.

Charles loved it because it was a buffet of spicy meats, vegetables, naan bread, and chutneys. I appreciated the wide variety of foods and my favorite, mango lassi. I still couldn't handle the meats, but I loved the smells and the ambiance. Charles got his plate, dove right in and ate to his heart's content. I was full after the lassi and sat back and watched him enjoy.

While we were dining, the numbness in my breast started to wear off. At first it felt like a dull ache, but it soon escalated to a steady throbbing. I went to the bathroom and looked at the area in the mirror. I couldn't see anything, but it was hurting. I went back to the table and told Charles we needed to leave. He hurriedly finished his Kheer.

By the time we got home, I wanted two pain pills, an ice bag, and my bed. I took off the bandage and looked at the place where the needle drilled into my skin to take a pinch of the mystery that lay beneath. It wasn't bleeding, but it was inflamed. The ice helped to cool it down. I waited for the medicine to relieve the pain.

Charles was at the end of the bed pacing back and forth. He wanted to do something, but there was nothing for him to do. He brought me more ice for the bag every fifteen minutes until we fell asleep.

The next morning, Charles was up and making breakfast. I was sore but didn't want to stay in bed, and it was too cold for any outside activities. My pain was now a dull ache. I cut back to one pain reliever and a hot pack. As I was taking the hot pack out of the microwave, my phone rang. I saw that it was a call from the Breast Cancer clinic and immediately grabbed the phone.

I recognized the voice of the nurse, "Mrs. Ross, we have the pathology report, and I have good news for you. There is no sign of cancer."

I had to let it sink in, so I said, "Would you repeat that?"

I could hear her smile as she repeated her good news.

"What was it?" I asked.

She explained that it was tissue calcification, which is normal in some post-menopausal women and scar tissue from a cyst that I had removed more than twenty years before. It had been so long ago, I forgot about the cyst.

Her last words were, "We will send you a report and see you in a year. Happy holidays to you and your family."

When Charles realized that I was talking to the nurse, he sat down across from me, and when I hung up, he could tell from my smile that it was good news. I forgot about my pain and made snacks while Charles set up the DVR and popped in the classic National Geographic documentary "Lions vs. Hyenas: Eternal Enemies."

While watching it, I thought about Us vs. Cancer.

Much like the lions, every time you think you've escaped the enemy, it might be lurking on the edges waiting to strike.

Christmas was a few weeks away. We went to a few parties, and I was ready to celebrate and have some fun. We didn't have much money, so I decided to make homemade desserts for gifts. I had much shopping to do because everyone wanted something different. Bria wanted a cheesecake, Brooke wanted creamy rice pudding with raisins, Stevie wanted a pound cake and sweet potato pie, Staci and Christian wanted oatmeal cookies.

I went to Brooke's house three days in a row to bake, and Kingston followed my every move. He was not allowed in the kitchen, so he stayed at the very edge of the room and watched. He was hoping for scraps, but since I was making desserts, I was reluctant to give him anything. Bria came home from school and informed me that he liked cookies. I made him some oatmeal cookies with bacon and less sugar.

I knew Daddy liked peanut brittle, and Mary liked boxed chocolate. Charles and I shopped for them and mailed our packages off to make sure they arrived a few days before Christmas. Skye was twenty-two months old and had every toy made for her age. I went shopping to buy her some clothes. I wanted to buy everything I saw from the pretty holiday dresses to the cute little jeans and tops for toddlers. Charles was picking up things and asking me how I thought she would look in it. We were enjoying ourselves and looked at this holiday with different eyes.

We all gathered at Brooke's home for Christmas dinner. I was happy to see Staci and Christian. It had been a while, and they were beaming about their recent engagement and wedding plans. Skye wanted us to see her Christmas Tree and all the lights. Bria showed us her new sneakers and cell phone.

After dinner, everyone wanted their gifts from me. Everyone opened their presents as if they were surprised, but a cake in a portable cake carrier or a pie wrapped in foil with a ribbon, or cookies in a holiday cookie tin with a snowman on it were thinly disguised at best and hardly surprising. I laughed out loud when Kingston came and sat beside me but wouldn't look at me. I went to the car and got his "special oatmeal cookies" that I put bacon bits in to make them more dog tasty. After I fed him a few of them, he turned his body to face me and laid over my feet.

It was a great day, and we all were looking forward to more days of peace, love, and family.

The new year was on the horizon, and I still didn't have an answer to the nagging question, "So what do you want to be now?"

I had a list of all the things I didn't want to be, however, discovery was not about elimination but possibilities. I wasn't yet sure what was possible.

With those feelings in mind and looking for direction, I went to church with Brooke and her family on New Year's Eve night to pray in the New Year. The service was set to begin at 10:00 p.m. and to end precisely at midnight. By the time we arrived at the church at 9:45, the pews were full. The ushers were asking everyone to squeeze in tight to make room for others. Brooke recognized one of her friends,

187

encouraging the people around her to make room so that we could sit near each other.

Two people refused to move, and I couldn't sit next to Brooke. Stevie was on duty as a "Peacekeeper." He stood at the side door to block entry from that area into the sanctuary.

Brooke was carrying Skye and Bria was carrying her diaper bag and books to keep her entertained until she fell asleep. As soon as we got settled, Skye cried out, "I want to be with Mema, I want to be with Mema!"

She crawled over people pushing and worming her way with the total freedom of a toddler until she landed in my lap with a thud.

She cried out again, "Bria, I want my book now."

Before she could turn around and head back, heads and hands turned to Bria and began passing the book to her.

She soon realized her power and simply said, "Sippy cup please," and the line fell into place.

The choir began to sing, and she sat up, clapped her hands, and tried to sing. When the pastor came to the podium to speak, she decided to grab my face and play with my earrings. She wanted to read her book to me, and when I told her not make noise, she started whispering the story in my ear. I was trying hard not to laugh and to pay attention to the words of inspiration from the pulpit. I was sure that she would get sleepy, but she was full of energy. Brooke signaled for me to send Skye back to her, but when I made a move, she yelled out "No, Mema, no!" and held on to my arm.

It was clear that she was taking control of the situation and that we were at her mercy. I can't remember what the sermon was about that night. I know what I learned from Skye: to ask for what you want, get others to help you do it, say please to those who help you, stop and enjoy the music, whisper when you can't speak loudly, say no when you feel like it and, above all, hold on.

HEALING BY
HELPING OTHERS

Charles was on his oral chemotherapy regime, some of his medications were reduced, and one eliminated. In late January, he came home from his appointment with a brochure for "Peer Partners" in big bold, blue letters. He handed it to me and asked me to read it and tell him what I thought.

Charles said, "Two ladies were recruiting for the program at Winship and I stopped by the table to get the information. I heard their presentation and thought it might interest you."

I was intently rushing to finish reading a book for my upcoming book club and put the brochure in the back of the book for later.

A few days later, I read it and it explained that a peer partner was a volunteer survivor or caregiver that would be matched to talk to a cancer patient or caregiver going through treatment with a similar cancer diagnosis. I was trying to get far away from cancer, only looking forward to when I could hear the words you have been cancer-free for five years, and you are CURED.

We agreed we wanted to volunteer and help in the community, but had very different thoughts about what we wanted to do. We decided that we didn't want to do it together and since we only had one car, and it was important that whatever we chose had to fit in with our gym and doctor's appointments.

Charles searched the internet for organizations that were seeking volunteers, and the list was overwhelming. There was the expected need to help feed the homeless and the unexpected need for volunteers to melt down used bar soap from hotels to be re-formed and packaged then donated to Third World countries. After two weeks of packaging soap, Charles decided it was not the best use of his time.

Next, he found an organization that collected books, sorted them by age group and subject, then boxed them to send to various villages in Africa for their schools. His heart was in it because of his memories of our trip to Africa. He saw the need, but the labor and conditions in the warehouse were not conducive to his immune system. So, after a month, he sadly told them goodbye. Before he left, someone gave him information on another organization.

This organization provided critical medical supplies and equipment to developing countries by recycling surplus materials from hospitals, U.S. manufacturers, and various healthcare systems.

The environment of the warehouse and the physical labor proved to be too much, and after six weeks, it too was over.

He landed at the Red Cross. The expansive organization seemed to be a perfect fit for any volunteer.

Charles found his passion for helping others and became a Disaster Relief Volunteer. Most calls were for fires, trees falling on houses, and floods.

He'd tell me about each event and seemed touched when there were children and pets involved.

I was visiting the Cancer center regularly and saw they were still recruiting for Peer Partners. After my appointment, I stopped and talked to the ladies named Julie and Linda. They were very friendly and outgoing. The more they talked, the more my perspective changed. Each shared stories from their several years as a volunteer.

We walked to the Patient and Family Resource Center, a quiet area that had information about specific cancers, support groups, social services. Patients and caregivers could sit in a relaxed area and have a respite between appointments. Linda led me to the office of a friendly woman named Davida, who was the manager of Volunteer Services.

She told me about the many ways I could use my experience and my talents to help others and their families. Her kind, gentle way and heartfelt appeal had me filling out forms in less than five minutes.

When I told Charles, he laughed, "My wife, you are one strong lady. Try as I might, I cannot walk back through those halls or visit the infusion center without breaking down."

I put my arms around him, "My husband, you are pretty amazing. I wouldn't attempt to go to a disaster and help people try to pick up tiny fragments of their lives while standing in rubble holding their children or an elderly parent."

Working with patients and their families is a significant responsibility. I was trained in what I could say, what I could do and where I could go if there were any problems. It was an honor to be trusted with the task and I took the opportunity to serve seriously. I remembered how kind and careful everyone was with Charles and me, and I wanted to do the same. My first goal was to stand before them as a survivor and offer them hope and my second was to listen to them and their caregiver or family member with an experienced ear that could say that not only do I understand, but also that I've been there.

The patients had familiar questions and requests. I found the striking differences were the caregivers. They were overwhelmed by the many tasks and expectations of caring for their loved one as well as children, husbands or wives, and other duties. A few of them left their jobs, and some left their families in other states to help a parent, sibling, or child.

The saddest cases were patients going through treatment alone; they had no family, or the family members chose not to be involved. It was heartbreaking to see how Cancer impacted areas of their lives that many people never talk about, well beyond the physical and financial.

I was a Peer Partner for six months when Davida asked me about serving on the Patient Family Advisory Council; I was humbled to be asked to serve on a committee that worked with doctors, staff, and on teams to collaborate on every aspect of patient and family care, except medical advice. The survivors that serve as PFA's are a caring group but also a force for change and have earned respect throughout the hospital.

Once a year in the fall, Winship held a 5K race to raise money for research and patient care. The second year after our treatment, Charles and I decided to start a team, which I named Ross ReMissionaries, since we were in remission. We raised money and had a small group of supporters. Charles won the second-place medal in his age group. His doctor was beaming as she stood with him and held his hand high. This was one more advancement in our new normal journey. With each step and stumble, we hoped we were moving in the right direction. We knew we had one more thing to do: a trip to Phoenix.

I called one of my friends, Tonya, and told her we were coming.

She said, "I want to throw you a party. Give me the names of your friends, former customers, and employees and I will take care of everything else."

We were excited to see the many people who wanted to see us. We had disappeared and never got to say goodbye to anyone, and we left them with many questions. As we flew into Phoenix, we recognized the Camelback in the distance. When we got out of the airport and took the first breath of the warm, dry air, we knew we were in familiar territory.

We arrived at the party a little late, but when someone saw us turn the corner, everyone poured out of the house, into the street and surrounded the car. When Charles unlocked the door, the crowd was pulling us out of our seats. There were touches, hugs, handshakes, kisses, squeals of delight, and tears. When we got into the house, more people were setting up tables and chairs and organizing the abundance of food and drinks that everyone contributed to.

Tonya's husband, who is a pastor, called everyone together to pray a prayer of Thanksgiving for our healing and our return. It was very moving and brought more tears. Charles spoke and thanked everyone as he told them about our journey. Someone turned on the music, and soon everyone was dancing, singing, and feasting in the warm Phoenix night.

We stayed for a week visiting old sights like our former restaurant and house. We saw other friends who were not at the party. We knew we would return to visit but not to live.

As we boarded the airplane, we looked at each other rising like the Phoenix bird from its ashes and, over our shoulders, we saw our fraternal twin Cancers going down in flames.

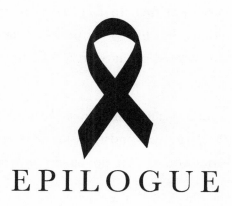

EPILOGUE

We continued to rebuild our life together sifting through the ashes looking for embers to spark a new flame.

I was passionate about working with cancer patients and caregivers and was spending an average of two days a week as a volunteer at Winship. Charles and I were featured in many ads and magazines. We traveled to Cincinnati to check on Dad after he was diagnosed with Parkinson's disease. Every two months when we visited him, he had lost another physical or mental function. I was heartbroken to see my Daddy diminished. It was like watching a fort being taken down, one brick at a time. My only consolation was Mary by his side like a dutiful soldier, making sure that the bricks were set aside with love and dignity. His final brick was laid to rest in January 2017.

In April 2018, Charles developed a cough and chest congestion which he attributed to seasonal allergies. Over the next month, his energy level bottomed out and he went to his primary care doctor who sent him for a chest x-ray that showed pneumonia in both lungs.

We weren't concerned at first. In fact, we were grateful it wasn't anything more serious. But his cough persisted, and he was losing weight. The doctor ordered a Cat Scan of his chest and called with the results.

"Mr. Ross, your scan indicates lung cancer. In your right lung in the upper lobe, there is a large mass and in the lower lobe, there is a smaller nodule. I am referring you to a Pulmonologist for further testing."

Charles was on the phone with the doctor when I walked in. I could see the blood draining out of his ashen and thinning face. I sat on the floor in front of him. He told me what the doctor said before retreating to the bedroom and closing the door.

I looked out of the window watching the beautiful sunny spring morning turn dark and foreboding.

My first emotion was anger. "Damn you Cancer, I believed you were gone. After eight years, here you are again. I'm not going to ask why. We are going to fight you with everything we've learned. You are sneaky, but I am not afraid."

Cancer stepped out of the shadows and into the sunlight, "Obviously you didn't learn very much because your doctors told you about recurrences and secondary cancers. If you think you can rise from the ashes now you see I can rise from the ashes of chemotherapy, radiation, and surgery. I don't need embers or new building blocks; I am now a part of you and your life, and I welcome the rematch."

I took a deep breath, said a short prayer, asked myself again,

"What do I want to be?"

198

The answer came from my soul, "A Warrior."

I must do whatever it takes to meet this without fear or doubt with what I learned in the first battle.

I checked on Charles and found him in the fetal position staring at the wall.

"Honey, we are going to fight this and win again. We are in a better position than before. We know lots of people at Winship, and they know us. We know that angels will come and some of the same ones will return. Once we let people know, the prayers will begin."

"Bari, please don't tell anyone. I don't want anybody to know except you, the doctors, and maybe Brooke."

I was stunned.

Cancer taunted me, "You didn't see that punch coming, did you? I claim round one and you just stepped in the ring."

I felt light-headed, but my determination was unwavering. I jetted over to the computer, printed the doctor's report, and read every word three times. I underlined and circled the things I didn't understand and highlighted the words that were familiar. Then I called to break the news to Brooke.

"Hi, Mommy. How are you doing, and how is Papa Charles?"

"His Cat Scan shows lung cancer and the doctor referred him to a Pulmonologist," I blurted out.

"What the what? I'm on my way over right now!"

I begged her not to come and promised to e-mail her a copy of the report.

Charles received a call from the Pulmonologist with an appointment for a biopsy. We were grateful how fast the hospital was responding.

I gave Brooke the appointment date.

"Whether he wants me to or not," she said, "I am coming to that appointment. I don't want you to assume anything until we get the results of the biopsy."

I breathed heavily as I felt the tears welling in my voice. It felt comforting to hear her say the same things she said almost nine years ago, and I relaxed in the familiar.

* * *

That night, as I wrestled with sleep, the word widow rang in my ears and flashed behind my closed eyes. I tried hard to push it away, but it persisted until I got up and began writing about what I thought it would mean to be a widow. Besides the obvious loss of my husband and the grieving, I began thinking about the impact such a loss would have on our family, our friends, and every aspect of my life. As determined as I was to fight, fear and doubt were creeping into my subconscious, and I knew that if I didn't meet it head on, it would immobilize me. I thought about the loneliness I would feel every day, the long days and nights without our funny banter or intense arguments, our incomplete "bucket list" of places we wanted to go and foods we wanted to try. I imagined how handicapped I would be driving at night with my terrible night vision. Charles drove us at night. My mind was flooded with thoughts of what losing my husband would mean. My sleep was a tangle of active nightmares and complete exhaustion.

***

The next morning, Charles was quiet while we ate our oatmeal, but every few minutes he would reach across the table and rub my hand.

"I know you asked me not to tell anyone, but I spoke to Brooke and sent her the report. She plans to go with us for the biopsy."

"Bari, I am glad you told Brooke. I don't want to burden her again with this but her knowledge and love for us is reassuring. I am embarrassed and ashamed to be in this position again. I feel like a loser. You know how hard we have worked to stay healthy. I eat right, I run every Saturday with my club, get my daily nap, I go to all doctor and dentist appointments, and yet here I am, facing cancer again."

I had no answers and fewer questions. I knew we had to play the hand we were dealt and hiding it from people was not a strong card if we were going to win.

***

I left for my water aerobics class hoping to distract my mind from all thing's cancer. That was not to be. As I approached the showers, I heard two women discussing and sharing their scarred chests from recent mastectomies. I turned my head to look away, but it was too late. I felt the punch in my stomach as Cancer strolled by and threw its fist in the air. I stepped into the fog of the steaming shower and let my tears mix with the water.

201

***

There was a sliver of light in the sky when Brooke arrived to take us to the hospital. Charles was solemn, but Brooke was a cheerleader, "Papa Charles, we got this. WE DID IT BEFORE. WE'LL DO IT AGAIN!"

In the waiting room, Brooke typed on her laptop as she listened on her earpiece. I forgot she was working remotely and had important reports and calls that needed handling while she helped us.

She removed her earpiece, "How are you, Mommy?"

"I'm ok. I think we both could use a cup of good coffee, and I could use some fresh air."

We walked across campus to her favorite Starbucks. As we sat there sipping our drinks, she got a beep from her laptop signaling an alert from her job. I sat back and watched her with admiration trying not to look through my mother eyes but woman to woman. She moved from one role to another seamlessly. It was nine-thirty in the morning and already it felt like a full day had passed.

When we stepped outside, the eighty-degree heat, the coffee, and the tension made me break out in a sweat. As I wiped my face, I glanced over at Brooke who was cool as an iced latte.

We returned to the waiting area and a nurse escorted us to a private room. A few minutes later the doctor came in.

"Mr. Ross tolerated the procedure well and is resting comfortably in post-op. I can't tell you exactly what he has, but I can tell you

202

I'm pretty certain it is not lung cancer. In my experience I have seen many lung cancers and the tissue does not look like any I've seen. I sent it to pathology, and we will wait for the results to discuss next steps. Do you have any questions?"

I wanted to hug the doctor but knew that wasn't proper. So, I hugged his words instead.

"Not lung cancer."

"Mommy, I told you to wait until after the biopsy to know whether it is lung cancer. This is great news. I'll call Steven and Staci while you go back and get him dressed so we can leave. I still have to get Skye from day camp and take her to swim practice."

I forgot about how Skye would fit into the day's schedule. As I walked down the hospital corridor toward Charles' room, I shook my head at the juggling act Brooke was performing.

I was surprised to find Charles sitting up in bed sipping cranberry juice and nibbling Lorna Doone cookies.

"Honey, the doctor said it's not lung cancer."

***

On the ride home, there was a livelier conversation filled with relief, joy, gratitude and one nagging question: What is it?

We were in an unsettled peace, waiting for the report. Charles' cough rattled in his chest and he would often fall asleep shortly after taking the medicine he was given. I was hesitant to leave him because sometimes the cough was so violent, it was disorienting. His

203

movements were weak, and I didn't want to risk a fall. Other times, I wanted to run out the door, drive four hours to the nearest beach, sit on a blanket facing the ocean, and scream at the waves.

Whenever his phone rang, I prayed it was his doctor with good news, but the calls were from telemarketers, unaware and uncaring of how they were intruding into our lives at the worst time.

***

Charles received a call from the doctor who treated him for Leukemia. Although I was in the kitchen, I could hear bits and pieces of the conversation he was having in the next room.

"That was Dr. A." Charles informed me as he hung up the phone and walked into the kitchen.

"She said the pulmonologist asked her to call me with the results. The best news is it is not lung cancer. The good news is it's not leukemia again. The bad news is that I have Hodgkin's Lymphoma. Dr. A says it is another blood cancer, but it is very treatable and curable with chemotherapy. She referred me to one of the hematologist-oncologists whose specialty is Lymphomas.

The key word was curable. We let out a sigh of relief and bumped fists.

Despite him not wanting to tell anyone, I felt I needed to tell someone in his family. I called Regenia and let her know Charles' desire to keep the news secret. She said it would be difficult, but she would respect his wishes.

While Charles slept, I slipped out for a long walk on a nearby trail. I passed the familiar pond full of late spring ducklings and baby geese being led by their cautious mothers. I walked slowly because it was the middle of the afternoon and it was hot, but also because I needed the time to breathe the fresh air. The air in our house was filled with cancer again and I needed to get out from under its dark wave, even if only for short time.

*   *   *

When I returned, Charles met me at the door,

"I heard from the doctor's office. I have appointments scheduled over the next few days"

At the first appointment, the nurse took Charles' vital signs and weight. He had lost fifteen pounds in six weeks. The doctor came in with a pleasant smile and hearty handshake.

She spoke briefly about his previous battle with leukemia and contrasted it with lymphoma. This lymphoma would not require him to spend weeks in the hospital or years on chemotherapy; instead, he would receive eight infusions over sixteen weeks.

The chemotherapy was a "cocktail" of four different medicines that were delivered through separate infusions over four or more hours. She would also prescribe medication to keep nausea at a minimum. She was certain that after the first treatment, his cough would diminish and after the second one, it would be gone.

Three days later, we were stepping through the doors of the infusion center.

The night before, I asked Charles his thoughts on going back.

"I am embarrassed to go back as a patient. I have spent the last year with patients and staff as an example of a fighter and survivor. I feel like I've let them down because I've got a second cancer. I don't know how they will feel, but I don't feel good about it."

I wanted to say, "Now you'll have a better and deeper story to tell about beating cancer twice."

I kept silent. We weren't there yet.

The next morning, we entered the lab. The staff recognized him. One person asked, "Mr. Charlie, what are you doing here—a regular check-up?"

He told her about his new diagnosis and her jaw dropped.

As we sat in the waiting room of the infusion center, Charles dozed lightly. I jostled him when I saw the volunteer with the hospitality cart approaching. When she reached us, he greeted her.

"Marybeth, it's me, Charlie, how are you?"

She was confused and disoriented by seeing him in the chair:

"Charlie, I thought you were on vacation or taking a break. Several of the patients have been asking for you. Why are you here?"

He told her what happened, and she sat down in the chair next to him. She said he would be in her prayers, grabbed the handle of the cart, and continued down the hall to serve others.

The nurse came to the door and invited us to follow her to the

206

treatment room. When Charles approached her, she stopped him,

"Mr. Charlie are you sure you are in the right place? Please, let me see your armband."

He explained everything to her. I saw her blinking back tears fighting to maintain her professionalism as she took his vitals.

As he rested in the infusion chair, a small parade of nurses, custodians, and volunteers came by to offer well wishes and prayers. He was like family to them and they wanted him to know his commitment to giving back and making a difference was appreciated.

We were talking when the nurse assigned to him approached the chair, busy reading the orders. He placed the papers on the standing desk and turned to introduce himself. As he extended his hand, he recognized Charles and his face and arm went limp. Charles spoke first.

"Daniel, yes it's me—Charlie the volunteer with the hospitality cart. You read the papers, so you know what's going on with me."

Daniel regained his composure and shook Charles' hand.

"I'm sorry that you are back here in the chair, but I promise you that the team and I will do everything we can to get you back behind the cart giving other patients hope with your story of beating cancer a second time."

Daniel began the first round of the "chemo cocktail." Charles' face flushed and his eyes rolled back. He took two deep breaths and on the third, he slumped and vomited into the can next to the chair.

Danny grabbed one of the now familiar green bags and handed it to Charles. He gave Charles more anti-nausea medicine and the rest of the "cocktail" went smoothly.

As the doctor promised, Charles' cough diminished after the first treatment, and at the end of the second, it was gone.

Staci came to Atlanta in July "to check on Charles," but it became apparent that it was a "Mommy check" as well. She made sure to take me to get a massage, manicure, and pedicure, as well as driving us to appointments and taking us out to lunch. She stayed for more than a week to let me, the weary caregiver, get a much-needed respite.

By the fifth round, Charles was feeling stronger and we started going for short walks. It was mid-August and he decided that he was going to participate in the October Winship 5K Run. He knew he wouldn't be able to run competitively but was sure he could at least walk the three miles.

A routine Pet Scan was scheduled shortly after Charles' seventh chemo treatment. He was feeling good and started to gain weight. We were walking two miles a day at least three days a week. We arrived at the doctor's office feeling confident. A young man entered the room, introduced himself as a resident, and assured us the doctor would be in shortly. He pulled up the initial scan and pointed to the right lung and we could see the area lit up like the Milky Way. I was stunned to see how invasive the tumor appeared. But when he pulled up the most recent scan, I was amazed when it showed no visible sign of the light that indicated the tumor.

Charles and I smiled at each other and I was about to throw up my hand for a high five when the resident said, "We aren't quite out of the woods yet. The radiologist sees a small shadow in the back of the lung, and we're obligated to let you know that you may need radiation after you complete your last chemotherapy."

I lowered my hand back in my lap. From the corner of my eye, I saw Cancer wink and disappear into the air. I looked at Charles and the hope and joy that was on his face a few seconds ago vaporized. In its place was a hint of disappointment and a flash of anger.

"I don't want radiation. I will take more chemo, but no radiation."

We sat there in stunned silence as we waited. We were used to being in this state, so neither of us bothered to try to fill the void with useless words. The doctor came through the door with her customary smile and headed for the hand sanitizer while simultaneously greeting Charles,

"I know my resident went over the scan with you and the current result isn't as definitive as we hoped. But I feel positive that the last chemo will clear everything that remains. It is a very small area, but we must be certain that there is no discernible cancer before we discontinue treatment. Radiation would be the next level of treatment, but let's wait until you complete your last chemo and I consult with the radiologist."

We agreed to take the information as a glancing blow rather than a knockout punch. We stopped and ate lunch at our favorite Indian restaurant. Over the chicken tikka masala, I said,

"Let's go for our walk later this evening and continue to train for the

209

5k. It's a month away and we've got to get up to three miles."

On October 13, 2018 surrounded by family and friends and many of the staff at Winship, we headed to the starting line hand in hand. It was a beautiful sunny day with the leaves on the trees dressed in bright oranges, reds and yellows swaying in a cool breeze. After the first mile, we let each other go. Charles walked ahead with Regenia and I trailed behind with Traci and Jerry. I kept my eye on him until he melted into the crowd. As Traci, Jerry, and I approached the finish line, we saw Charles and Reginia holding the white carnations that are presented to survivors. When I received mine, I went over to my husband and presented it to him because he fought this dreaded disease twice and I believed he won.

Two weeks later, it was confirmed. The doctor walked into the room with a big smile on her face, "Mr. Ross, there is no sign of cancer anywhere. You are cured. There will be no radiation. I'll see you in three months for a check-up."

He hugged her, "Thank you. Thank you for all your hard work."

* * *

Once again, we are looking toward the future. In a few months, Charles will return to the hospitality cart and what a story he will share with those he serves and those who served him in the infusion center.

I continue to volunteer and advocate for cancer patients.

I heard a speaker say, "Cancer is a disease that takes far too much from far too many in this day and time."

I know it is true through our experience, through people I talk to, and the initiatives I work with. I try not to look over myshoulder for the specter of Cancer, but time and time again it reveals its sinister shadow through a call or an encounter that begins with three words, "I have cancer."

Despite the growing number of cancer cases, the fastest growing number is the number of survivors.

We are blessed to be counted as survivors.